first place 4 health

bible study series

begin with Christ

Published by Gospel Light
Ventura, California, U.S.A.
www.gospellight.com
Printed in the U.S.A.

Caution: The information contained in this book is intended to be solely for informational and educational purposes. It is assumed that the First Place 4 Health participant will consult a medical or health professional before beginning this or any other weight-loss or physical fitness program.

Library of Congress Cataloging-in-Publication Data
First Place 4 health Bible study #1: Begin with Christ.
p. cm.
ISBN 978-0-8307-4518-0 (trade paper)
1. Bible—Study and teaching. 2. Christian life—Study and teaching.
I. Title: First Place for health Bible study.
BS600.3.F57 2008
242'.5—dc22
2008000345

contents

foreword

My introduction to Bible study came when I joined First Place in March 1981. I had been attending church since I was a small child, but the extent of my study of the Bible had been reading my Sunday School quarterly on Saturday night. On Sunday morning, I would listen to my Sunday School teacher as she taught God's Word to me. During the worship service, I would listen to our pastor as he taught God's Word to me. Frankly, digging out the truths of the Bible for myself had never entered my mind.

Perhaps you are right where I was back in 1981. If so, you are in for a blessing you never dreamed possible. As you start studying the truths of the Bible for yourself through the First Place 4 Health Bible studies, you will see God begin to open your understanding of His Word.

Almost every First Place 4 Health member I have talked with about the program says, "The weight loss is wonderful, but the most important thing I have received from my association with First Place 4 Health is learning to study God's Word." The First Place 4 Health Bible studies are designed to be done on a daily basis. As you work thorough each day's study (which will take 15 to 20 minutes to complete), you will be discovering the deep truths of God's Word. A part of each week's study will also include a Bible memory verse for the week.

There are many in-depth Bible studies on the market. The First Place 4 Health Bible studies are not designed for the purpose of in-depth study, but are designed to be used in conjunction with the rest of the program to bring balance into your life. Our desire is for each member to begin having a personal quiet time with God each day. This time alone with God should include a time of prayer, Bible reading and Bible study. Having a quiet time is a daily discipline that will bring the rich rewards of balance, which is something we all need.

God bless you as you begin this exciting journey toward a balanced life. God will richly bless your efforts to give Him first place in your life. Remember Matthew 6:33: "But seek first his kingdom and his righteousness, and all these things will be given to you as well."

Carole Lewis
First Place National Director

introduction

First Place 4 Health is a Christ-centered health program that emphasizes balance in the physical, mental, emotional and spiritual areas of life. The First Place 4 Health program is meant to be a daily process. As we learn to keep Christ first in our lives, we will find that He is the One who satisfies our hunger and our every need.

This Bible study is designed to be used in conjunction with the First Place 4 Health program but can be beneficial for anyone interested in obtaining a balanced lifestyle. The Bible study has been created in a five-day format, with the last two days reserved for reflection on the material studied. Keep in mind that the ultimate goal of studying the Bible is not only for knowledge but also for application and a changed life. Don't feel anxious if you can't seem to find the *correct* answer. Many times, the Word will speak differently to different people, depending on where they are in their walk with God and the season of life they are experiencing. Be prepared to discuss with your fellow First Place 4 Health members what you learned that week through your study.

There are some additional components included with this study that will be helpful as you pursue the goal of giving Christ first place in every area of your life:

- **Group Prayer Request Form:** This form is at the end of each week's study. You can use this to record any special requests that might be given in class.

- **Leader Discussion Guide:** This discussion guide is provided to help the First Place 4 Health leader guide a group through this Bible study. It includes ideas for facilitating a First Place 4 Health class discussion for each week of the Bible study.

- **First Place 4 Health Menu Plans**: There are 14 days of meals, and all are interchangeable. Each day totals 1,400 to 1,500 calories and includes snacks. Instructions are given for those who need more calories. An accompanying grocery list includes items that will be needed for each week of meals.

- **First Place 4 Health Member Survey:** Fill this out and bring to your first meeting. This information will help your leader know your interests and talents.
- **Personal Weight and Measurement Record:** Use this form to keep a record of your weight loss. Record any loss or gain on the chart after the weigh in at each week's meeting.
- **Weekly Prayer Partner Forms:** Fill out this form before class and place it into a basket during the class meeting. After class, you will draw out a prayer request form, and this will be your prayer partner for the week. Try to call or email the person sometime before the next class meeting to encourage that person.
- **Live It Trackers:** Your Live It Tracker is to be completed at home and turned in to your leader at your weekly First Place 4 Health meeting. The Tracker is designed to help you practice mindfulness and stay accountable with regard to your eating and exercise habits. Step-by-step instructions for how to use the Live It Tracker are provided in the *Member's Guide*.
- **Let's Count Our Miles!** A worthy goal we encourage is for you to complete 100 miles of exercise during your 12 weeks in First Place 4 Health. There are many activities listed on pages 255-256 that count toward your goal of 100 miles. When you complete a mile of activity, mark off the box listed on the chart located on the inside of the front cover.
- **Scripture Memory Cards:** These cards have been designed so that you can use them while exercising. It is suggested that you punch a hole in the upper left corner and place the cards on a ring. You may want to take the cards in the car or to work so that you can practice each week's Scripture memory verse throughout the day.
- **Scripture Memory CD:** All 10 Scripture memory verses have been put to music at an exercise tempo in the CD at the back of this study. Use this CD when exercising or even when you are just driving in your car. The words of Scripture are often easier to memorize when accompanied by music.

Use each of these important tools found in this study to live a balanced and healthy life.

Week One

welcome to *Begin with Christ*

Congratulations! And welcome to the First Place 4 Health *Begin with Christ* Bible study. We are so glad you have chosen to join us on this lifelong journey to health, wholeness and a balanced lifestyle that honors God.

At your first group meeting for this session of First Place 4 Health, you will meet your fellow members, get an overview of your materials and find out what you can expect at weekly meetings. The majority of your class time will be spent learning about the four-sided person concept, the Live It Food Plan, and how change begins from the inside out. You will also have a chance to ask any questions about how to get the most out of First Place 4 Health. If possible, complete the Member Survey on page 205 before your first group meeting. The information you give will help your leader tailor the next 12 weeks to the needs of the whole group.

Each weekly meeting begins with a weigh-in for members. This will allow you to track your progress over the 12-week session. Your Week One weigh-in/measurement will establish a baseline of comparison so that you can set healthy goals for this session. If you are apprehensive about weighing in every week, talk with your group leader about your concerns. He or she will have some options for you to consider that will make the weigh-in activity encouraging rather than stressful.

The day after your first meeting, begin Week Two of this Bible study. This session, you and your group will explore the importance of centering your goals for a healthy life on Jesus. No matter how strong your body, mind and emotions may appear, unless you have spiritual tenacity and resolve, you will not be able to run the course God has laid out before you. As you open yourself to the truth of Scripture and share your hopes and struggles with the members of your group during the next 12 weeks, you'll find yourself becoming the healthy child of God you are designed to be!

Week Two

getting to know Him

Scripture Memory Verse

Seek first his kingdom and his righteousness, and all these things will be given to you as well.

Matthew 6:33

In choosing First Place 4 Health, you have made a decision that has life-changing potential. Our Creator fashioned us as multi-faceted beings: people with a wonderfully made body, an intricate mind, a wide range of emotions–and a spiritual dimension, too. That's why only a program that addresses our needs on all four levels has the ability to cure the angst that keeps us from realizing our health and fitness goals.

Proverbs 24:10 gives us some wise counsel that will help us realize the importance of being steadfast in body, mind, emotions and spirit: "If you falter in times of trouble, how small is your strength!" If we concentrate all of our effort on just the physical aspect of health and wholeness, we will surely falter when the road gets difficult and we are faced with temptation. No matter how strong our bodies, minds and emotions may appear, unless we have spiritual tenacity and resolve, we will not be able to run the course God has laid out before us. Likewise, if we concentrate all our effort on gaining spiritual strength but neglect the precious body God has entrusted to our care, our lack of physical discipline, emotional self-control and mental perseverance will be our undoing. Only a health and fitness program that brings balance to our four-sided being can restore us to the health and wholeness that honors our Creator.

As we begin this study, take a moment to complete an honest assessment of where you are with regard to strength, stamina and stability in each of the four aspects of your being. This will help you identify your weak areas, those parts you need to shore up until you have increased your strength. The assessment will also help you identify your strengths: the areas that will be the mainstays of your First Place 4 Health program while you grow and develop the areas that are currently frail. In doing this evaluation, remember that this exercise is not an occasion to belittle or berate yourself. This is strictly diagnostic information—information you can utilize when times of temptation come. By knowing where you are strong and where you are weak, you will be better able to protect yourself. Having identified your strengths and weaknesses, you will be able to lead from your strengths rather than putting excess pressure on areas that are more vulnerable. Rate yourself on a scale from 1 to 5, with 1 being the weakest and 5 the strongest:

Physical Strength, Stamina and Stability	1	2	3	4	5
Emotional Strength, Stamina and Stability	1	2	3	4	5
Mental Strength, Stamina and Stability	1	2	3	4	5
Spiritual Strength, Stamina and Stability	1	2	3	4	5

Carefully assess your answers. We will revisit this diagnostic tool at the end of our *Begin with Christ* Bible study so that you can praise God for the progress you have made during this 12-week segment of our ongoing effort to put Christ first in all things.

THE SUPREMACY OF CHRIST

Day 1

Almighty God, in You are hidden all the treasures of wisdom and knowledge. As I begin this Bible study, I pray that You will open my spiritual eyes so that I can see You in new and exciting ways. By the power of Your Holy Spirit, please give me the grace to clearly understand and freely choose the way of Your wisdom through Christ my Lord. Amen.

It is one thing to say that Christ has first place in our life; it is quite another to put those words into practice. But before we can say that Christ has authority in our life, it is important that we understand who this Christ is that we are turning our life and will over to! Faith cannot be confused with foolishness. Part of our problem in the past has been foolishly putting our trust in people and programs that were not worthy of our confidence. So during this week of our *Begin with Christ* Bible study, we are going to learn more about Jesus, the One who is altogether faithful and completely worthy of our trust.

The apostle Paul presents us with a very detailed description of the work and ministry of Jesus Christ. Turn to Colossians 1:15-20 in your Bible, and then read Paul's description. What do you learn about Jesus Christ in these verses?

Jesus is God

You may want to reread Paul's words so that you can grasp the entire truth presented in this passage. Verse 18 tells us:

> And he is the head of the body, the church; he is the beginning and the firstborn from among the dead, so that in everything he might have the supremacy.

Having read Paul's words, rewrite the passage in your own words, substituting "first place" for the word "supremacy."

We should give Jesus Christ first place in our lives because he is the prince of peace. He is the Lord of All.

After meditating on Colossians 1:15-20, what new information about Jesus Christ did you learn that will make you more inclined to surrender your life and will to this man called Jesus the Christ? Be specific and list as many new facts as the Holy Spirit impressed upon your heart during this reading.

Just prior to the passage we have been studying today, Paul gives us another important fact about Jesus. Read Colossians 1:10-14. What has Christ done for you that assures you of a place in God's kingdom and qualifies you to share in the inheritance of the saints in the kingdom of light?

God sent Jesus to rescue us from darkness, so that our sins can be forgiven.

How is First Place 4 Health part of "growing in the knowledge of God" and "being strengthened with all power according to his glorious might so that you may have great endurance and patience" (verses 10-11)?

Learn to pray for others

In verse 10, Paul prays that those reading his words would "live a life worthy of the Lord and . . . please him in every way." How is Paul's prayer related to this week's Scripture memory verse?

If we seek the Kingdom of God and his rightous we will please God, bear good fruit, grow in the knowledge of God, and be filled with God's strenght.

Gracious God, I am humbled when I read of who Jesus Christ is and what He has done for me. Help me to apply the words of today's study to my life so that I can grow in the knowledge of God and be strengthened in the core of my spiritual being. Amen.

THEN AND NOW

Day 2

Prepare my heart, O God, to accept Your Word. Silence in me any voices but Your own so that I may clearly hear what You want to teach me today in and through Christ my Lord. Amen.

Yesterday we studied Paul's wonderful words about the work and ministry of Jesus Christ as described in Colossians 1:10-20. As we begin today's study, recap what you learned yesterday, especially as it applies to your participation in First Place 4 Health.

Jesus Christ is God/He rescued us from Satan/Made us his children/brought us into his eternal life/he redeemed us and forgave us all from sin

In order to fully appreciate what Christ has done for us, it is important that we acknowledge what our life was like before Christ appeared to us. Turn to Titus 3:3-5 in your Bible, and prayerfully read the passage.

In verse 3, Paul tells us what our life was like "at one time." Although these words could be applied to many areas of our life, today we are going to apply them to our health and fitness efforts. How were you deceived and enslaved by the diet and exercise programs you tried in the past?

Did not have the control to stop from eating things which I desired.

What kinds of passions and pleasures ruled your life before Jesus Christ set you free? Make your answer applicable to those things that kept you from achieving your health and fitness goals.

Eating Sweets

How did your chronic lack of loving self-care contribute to malice and envy, especially envy of those who took good care of themselves?

Sometimes it made me eat more

Titus 3:4-5 contains a precious truth. Read these verses carefully. You might even want to underline them in your Bible! Who appeared, and what did He do? Paraphrase Titus 3:4-5 in your own words.

We move from a life full of sin to one where we are led by God's Holy Spirit. Are sins are all washed away.

What had you done to deserve God's kindness and love?

Nothing. It is God's gift.

If you had done nothing righteous (that is, nothing to make yourself right with God), why did God your Savior appear?

A Gift because he loves us.

What additional information have you learned about Jesus Christ after completing today's lesson?

Jesus will be with me all the way.
In everything I do.

After contemplating what Jesus Christ did for you, you are undoubtedly overflowing with gratitude that you need to turn into jubilant praise. Write a letter expressing your thankfulness to the One who saved you because of His great mercy. Record your letter below, or use your spiritual journal to record your prayer of thanksgiving.

Dear Father thank you so much for
Showing mercy on me.. Thank you for
your undying Love.

Almighty and merciful God, thank You for Jesus. When I was lost He saved me, not because of any good thing I had done, but because of Your great mercy and love. Amen.

A GREAT HIGH PRIEST

Day 3

Gracious God, today I pray You will give me a humble, teachable and obedient heart so that I may receive the truth You will reveal to me in today's lesson; and that I may then put that lesson into practice in my life. Amen.

Not only did Jesus, the One we are learning more about this week, save us when we were deceived and enslaved, but He also continues to play a vital role in our efforts to live a life pleasing to God. Turn to Hebrews 4:14-16 in your Bible.

According to verse 14, what role does Jesus Christ play in our twenty-first-century lives?

Jesus was tempted, the same way we
are tempted today.

How does the fact that Jesus is our "great high priest" benefit us (verse 14)?

Because we want to be like Jesus.
He was without sin and we need to
follow him.

Verse 15 tells us that there is something unique about this great high priest. What makes Jesus Christ different from the priests who ministered to God's people before Christ came to save us from our sins?

Because he was tempted and without sin.

Jesus, our high priest, was tempted in every way, just as we are! He will never chide or scold us when we come to Him in our weakness. Verse 16 tells us about a very special benefit of having Jesus as our high priest. What is that benefit?

Confidence to help us.

According to verse 16, what do we receive when we come to God in our time of need?

Confidence

Reflecting on the inventory you did at the beginning of this week's study, what personal vulnerabilities do you need to bring to Jesus so that He can shore up your weakness with His strength?

Temptation

How is doing a daily First Place 4 Health Bible study that is specifically designed to increase spiritual strength and stamina an essential part of holding firmly to the faith you profess?

Jesus Christ will always be there for us.

How is caring for the other three aspects of your being—your body, your mind and your emotions—part of holding firmly to the faith you profess?

Because Jesus will always be there for us.

According to Proverbs 24:10, which we read in the introduction to this week's study, what happens to us during times of temptation when we are not strong in equal measure in body, mind, emotions and spirit?

We will not be able to stay ontrack.

How is First Place 4 Health helping you to overcome your weaknesses through the power of Jesus Christ, your Lord?

Because I know Jesus was tempted & I will try harder.

Thank You, God, for giving me a great high priest who can sympathize with my weakness. Because He was tempted as I am, I can come to You for grace and help, no matter how weak and helpless I may feel. Amen.

I AM

Day 4

O Lord, I do not live by bread alone but by every word that comes from Your mouth. Make me hunger for this heavenly food, that it may nourish me today. I ask this in the name of Jesus, the bread that came down from heaven. Amen.

So far we have been looking at what other people have said about Jesus. Today we are going to learn what Jesus said about Himself. The Gospel of John gives us some "I Am" statements Jesus made. Who did Jesus say He was?

John 6:48: "I am the bread of life."

John 8:12: "I am the light of the world."

John 8:23: "I am from above."

John 10:9: "I am the gate."

John 10:11: "I am the good sheppard."

John 10:36: "I am God's Son."

John 11:25: "I am the surrectron and the life."

John 14:6: "I am the way, and the truth, and the life."

John 15:1: "I am the true vine."

John 18:37: "I am a King."

What do these "I Am" statements teach you about Jesus that you did not learn about Him in our Day One, Day Two or Day Three study?

Jesus is everywhere.

Reread the list of "I Am" statements you have just compiled. Ask the Holy Spirit to show you which "I Am" statement you most need to believe today so that you will be better prepared to surrender your life and will to the Lordship of Jesus Christ. Which verse did you pick, and why?

I am the way, and the truth and the life. Because I always want to follow God, and I know the truth will set me free.

Finally, let's read what God the Father has to say about Jesus, His Son. Turn to Mark 9:7 in your Bible. What does God say about Jesus?

This is my son, whom I Love. Listen to him.

How is listening to Jesus, God's beloved Son, part of your First Place 4 Health program, and why?

Because we need spiritual guidance to achieve good health.

Loving and gracious Lord, You are the way, the truth and the life. Help me to listen carefully to everything You say, knowing that You and You alone can satisfy my hungry soul. Amen.

MY LORD AND MY GOD

Day 5

May the words of my mouth and the meditation of my heart be pleasing in your sight, O LORD, my Rock and my Redeemer. Amen (Psalm 19:14).

After His cruel death on the cross at Calvary, Jesus rose from the tomb and appeared to His disciples before He ascended back to the right hand of His Father. One disciple, Thomas, was not with the others when Jesus first appeared to them. Later, when Thomas was in their midst, Jesus reappeared. Turn to John 20:24-25 in your Bible, and read about the beginning of the incident.

What did Thomas say to the other disciples about believing that Jesus had risen from the dead (verse 25)?

He needed to see Jesus and put his finger through the nail holes,

Now read John 20:26-27. What was Jesus' greeting to the disciples when He entered the house (verse 26)?

Peace Be With You

Was Thomas at peace when Jesus first came into the room? Explain your answer.

He was doubting Jesus.

Even though Jesus had not been in the room when Thomas declared he would not believe unless he saw the nail marks and put his hand into Jesus' side, Jesus knew exactly what was keeping Thomas from believing He was the risen Christ. What did Jesus say to Thomas (verse 27)?

Put you finger here, see my hands. Reach out your hand and put it into my side.

According to verse 28, what was Thomas's response?

My Lord and my God

Jesus also knows exactly what is keeping you from truly believing that He is the risen Christ. What does Jesus need to do to convince you that He is the One who died for your sins and deserves supremacy in your life? Spend some time today talking to Jesus about your doubts and fears and your questions and anxieties. Record this conversation below—or better yet, in your spiritual journal.

When you have finished writing, hear your Lord say, "Peace be with you!" He will prove Himself worthy of the title "My Lord and My God," if you will only give Him an opportunity to do so. But you must also do your part. Reread Jesus' words to Thomas. What is Jesus saying to you through this account?

Never Doubt and always believe.

How can First Place 4 Health help you stop doubting and start believing?

Praying for everyone will bring me closer to God.

When you, along with Thomas, can boldly declare, "My Lord and my God," you will be ready to put Christ first in all things. What is standing between you and making that bold confession right now?

Finding time

Once that obstacle is removed, what will keep you from caring for your body, mind, emotions and spirit in a way that reflects God's great love for you in Christ Jesus, your Lord and your God? Be specific in your answer.

I work 10 hrs a day. Take care of a husband for suffers from Depression. Two parents in the hospital.

My Lord and my God, thank You for showing Yourself to me in ways that calm my anxious fears. Thank You for appearing and reappearing until I can finally grasp the height, breadth, depth and width of Your love for me. Amen.

REFLECTION AND APPLICATION

Day 6

O Lord, Your Word is a lamp to my feet and a light for my path. Give me the grace to receive your truth in faith and love, and the strength to follow the path you set before me, through Jesus Christ. Amen (Psalm 119:105).

During our Day Four study, we looked at 10 "I Am" statements made by Jesus Christ. One day while Jesus and His disciples were alone, Jesus asked them, "Who do the crowds say I am?" (Luke 9:18). In response to Jesus' question, the disciples answered, "Some say John the Baptist, others say Elijah; and still others, that one of the prophets of long ago has come back to life" (Luke 9:19). Having heard their answer, Jesus then asked His disciples a piercing question, the same piercing question He is asking you today: "But what about you? . . . Who do you say I am?" Simon Peter boldly declared, "The Christ of God" (Luke 9:20).

Reflecting on what you have learned during this week of the *Begin with Christ* Bible study, write 10 "You Are" statements in response to Jesus' question "Who do you say I am?" Don't just paraphrase Jesus' "I Am" statements, but rather search your heart and write a genuine confession of your belief in Jesus, the Christ of God.

You are the father of the universe

You are our salvation

You are the beginning + the end

You are good Shepperd

You are my friend

You are the Son of God

You are eternal life

You are my listening Box

You are Love

You are peace

Having declared who Jesus is, go about your day so that your very life becomes a tribute to the One who saved you because of His great mercy.

O Lord God Almighty, You are the Son of God, the One who came to save me from my sins. Thank You for revealing Yourself to me through the Begin with Christ Bible study. The more I know You, the more I love You. Thank You for calling me to be one of Your disciples and for allowing me to sit at Your feet and learn from You. Amen.

Day 7

REFLECTION AND APPLICATION

My Lord and my God, You are the source of all light; through Your Word, You give light to my soul. Pour out on me the spirit of wisdom and understanding that my heart and mind may be opened to Your truth. Amen.

This week you have discovered many truths about Jesus Christ, the One who saved you because of His great mercy. Before going on to the Week Three study, spend some time today allowing the truths you have learned this week to soak into the depth of your being. Perhaps your spiritual muscles are even a bit sore, much like your physical muscles are sore when you first begin to exercise! And just as you might soak your aching physical muscles in a hot tub or spa, soak your aching spiritual muscles in the warmth and love of God's Word.

Reflect on the truths about Jesus that you have learned during Week Two of *Begin with Christ*. What truth was new information, something you had not realized about Jesus before now?

What truth that you have known for some time was reaffirmed or presented in a way that shed new light on your commitment to Jesus?

If Jesus were in the room with you right now, what question would you ask Him that would help you believe and not doubt? By the power of the Holy Spirit, Jesus is closer to you than your own breath, so why don't you pick up your spiritual journal and spend some time asking Jesus to encourage and strengthen your heart? Pause as you write so that Jesus can talk to you, too! Remember that this is the Son of God speaking, and you are to listen to Him!

> *O gracious and loving Lord, thank You for revealing Yourself to me so that I can grow in grace and knowledge of You. You are my Lord and my God, and it is my desire to please You in all that I do. Today I surrender my will and my way to Your Lordship, especially as it applies to caring for my body, mind, heart and spirit as a reflection of Your great love for me. Amen.*

Group Prayer Requests

first place 4 health

Today's Date: ________________

Name	Request

Results

____

____

____

____

____

____

____

Week Three

pray for spiritual stamina and strength

SCRIPTURE MEMORY VERSE
If you believe, you will receive whatever you ask for in prayer.
MATTHEW 21:22

Last week's *Begin with Christ* Bible study introduced us to Jesus, the One we strive to put first in all things. In order to love and serve Him, it is essential that we know who He is! We do not serve an unknown god; we worship and adore the almighty sovereign Lord, a God who is eager to reveal Himself, a God who invites us to seek Him with all our heart, mind, body and spirit (see Mark 12:30; Luke 10:27). He loves us with an everlasting love and longs to be in an intimate relationship with us much more than we desire to be close to Him! His door is always open to us (see Matthew 7:7). As we learned last week, because Jesus is our great high priest, we can approach God with bold confidence, knowing we will receive grace and help in our time of need.

Getting to know God by studying a portion of God's Word each day is an important aspect of our success in First Place 4 Health; however, simply reading the Bible is not enough to establish an ongoing relationship with the Master we serve. Daily communication with God through prayer is essential if we are going to build spiritual strength, stamina and stability.

We see an example of the importance of getting to know Jesus on a personal level in John 4:39-42. We are told that a group of Samaritans wanted to see Jesus because they heard about Jesus from a woman Jesus had talked to beside a well. Because of what the woman said to them, they wanted to know more about this man called Jesus who claimed to have living water. After a personal encounter with the living Lord, they declared, "We no longer believe just because of what you said; now we have heard for ourselves, and we know that this man really is the Savior of the world" (verse 42). And so it is with us.

We can listen to the words of others about Jesus, but in order to know that He is really our Lord and Savior, we must personally encounter the living Lord. Secondhand knowledge is never a substitute for firsthand faith.

Bible study and prayer are to spiritual fitness what aerobic exercise and strength training are to physical fitness. It takes both, working in tandem, to develop strength, endurance and stability. Our God is not far off and detached from His chosen people. As a matter of fact, the Christ we worship and serve wants to be intimately involved in every aspect of our being—even in seemingly insignificant things like what we eat and how we care for our body, mind, heart and spirit. Acts 17:28 tells us an essential truth: "In Him we live and move and have our being."

Day 1

THE DAILY DISCIPLINE OF PRAYER

O Lord, today I pray for eyes to see, ears to hear and a heart to receive the truth You want to teach me in today's lesson. Jesus sent the Holy Spirit to lead me into all truth. Today I pray for the Spirit's guidance, in Jesus' name. Amen.

It has been said that if Christians prayed half as much as they worry, soon they would have nothing to worry about! As we begin today's Bible study, stop for a moment and recall the number of times this week that you worried about your health and fitness: what you were going to eat, how your body looked, what your body image said about you, or how you were going to conceal the excess pounds and inches you wear underneath your outer clothing. How many hands would you need to count the number of times you worried?

Now turn to Matthew 6:25-32 in your Bible. What did Jesus have to say about worry, especially as it applies to what we eat and what we wear?

Do not worry

Jesus asked His disciples a question about what worry can accomplish (verse 27). Answer that question as though you are replying directly to Jesus.

According to verse 30, Jesus made a statement about those who worry about what they will eat and what they will wear:

O you of little faith.

Are those His words to you today? Why or why not?

Yes, because God will provide for us. We need a always have faith and trust God.

How is worry like doubting (having little faith), and what is God's kingdom solution to both worry and unbelief? (It is the focal point of this week's Bible study!)

Our memory verse for last week (Matthew 6:33) was part of Jesus' teaching about not worrying about tomorrow. By way of review, write down last week's memory verse.

Seek first His Kingdom and His righteousness and all these things will be given to you as well.

Earlier in Matthew 6, Jesus had given His disciples a prayer in response to their request that He teach them to pray. After instructing His disciples to acknowledge who God is and to pray for the coming of God's kingdom here on Earth, Jesus told the disciples to pray for their physical needs. Read Matthew 6:11. What exact words did Jesus use?

Give us today our daily bread.

Go back to the sentence you wrote above and underline the word "daily." Now read Matthew 6:34, the conclusion of the passage we have been studying today. How does Matthew 6:34 affirm what Jesus said in Matthew 6:11?

Rather than worrying about tomorrow, what did Jesus tell His followers to do?

Plan for tomorrow.
Living one day at a time keeps us from being consumed with worry.

What have Jesus' words taught you about the need for daily prayer?

We must pray to God for our daily needs and trust God will take care of us.

Father, thank You that You have promised to provide for my daily needs if I will only come to You in prayer, asking for my daily bread. Today I will use my time to pray, not worry, confident that You know what I need before I even ask! Amen.

Day 2

CASTING YOUR CARES

O Lord God, You are the One who daily bears my burdens. Today give me the grace to cast my worries and fears upon You, confident that when I do so, You will lift me up and restore me to vibrant spiritual health. Amen.

During yesterday's *Begin with Christ* study, we learned about the importance of replacing worry with prayer. But if we are not to worry, exactly what are we to do with the cares that keep us burdened physically, mentally, emotionally and spiritually? Those of us who have spent a lifetime worrying about many things know that our worries don't just magically disappear! We need to have a place to put our anxious concerns before we can fold our hands in prayer. As always, our gracious God, the One who knows what we need before we even ask, gives us the ideal solution to the "what to do with our worries" dilemma.

Turn to 1 Peter 5:6-9 in your Bible. What are the four instructions given by the apostle Peter at the beginning of each verse?

Verse 6:

Humble yourselves under Gods mighty hand

Verse 7:

Cast all you anxiety on God

Verse 8:

Be self controlled and alert

Verse 9:

Stand firm in the feith of God

What does God promise to do when we humble ourselves under His mighty hand (verse 6)?

He will lift us up.

How is praying rather than worrying part of humbling ourselves under God's almighty hand? Carefully think about this question, remembering that one aspect of humility is complete dependence on God.

Verse 7 instructs us to cast our anxiety on God. Why are we instructed to do this?

Because God will help us bear the weight.

How is God's request that we cast our cares on Him because He cares for us part of God's provision for all our daily needs?

Trust

When you cast your cares on God, what happens to your anxiety and fear?

He helps us bear them.

The psalmist confidently declared, "Praise be to the Lord, to God our Savior, who daily bears our burdens" (Psalm 68:19). What do these words teach you about the need to cast your cares on God at the beginning of every day?

Trust God everyday.

Look again at 1 Peter 5. Verse 8 instructs us to be in control of ourselves and to be always watchful. Reflect on a time when you were worried and anxious—neither self-controlled nor alert. What happened? How were your eating habits affected? The benefit of allowing God to daily bear our burdens is listed in verse 8. How does casting your cares onto God's broad shoulders allow you to be self-controlled and alert? Once again, give this question careful thought. Perhaps you would like to reflect back to a time when you were worried and anxious, and neither self-controlled nor alert, before you answer.

According to 1 Peter 5:8, who is at the root of our anxiety and unbelief?

Satan

How do anxiety and unbelief devour us?

Over eating.

As compulsive eaters, what might we devour when we are worried and anxious?

Cookies

First Peter 5:9 tells us how to handle this ancient foe. What are we instructed to do?

Resist, stand firm in the faith.

How are First Place 4 Health and the daily discipline of prayer part of standing firm in your faith when you find yourself under enemy attack?

Because God will help me overcome.

Verses 10-11 of 1 Peter 5 outline the marvelous blessing we receive when we cast our cares onto God because He cares for us. Read these words prayerfully, and then continue in prayer as you thank God for restoring you and making you strong, firm and steadfast. You might want to record your thank-You prayer in your spiritual journal.

Thank You, gracious Father. You are the One who restores my weary soul when it is burdened with the cares of this world. O Lord, please forgive me for the times I worry rather than pray. Help me to stand firm in my faith, confident that You care for me. Amen.

Day 3

WHAT GOD ASKS OF YOU

Gracious and loving Father, all too often I make following Your will difficult instead of simply doing what You ask of me. Help me to see the truth in today's lesson so that I can apply it to my life. Amen.

Often we make what God asks of us very complex when, in truth, our gracious God gives us simple instructions—things that are not too difficult or beyond our reach. Micah 6:6-8 is one of God's simple instruction passages. Turn to it now, and carefully read what God requires of you.

This passage begins with a series of questions about what we must do to please God. How might the foolish diet and exercise programs we have turned to in the past be akin to these questions? Read the words over again, and then be creative in your explanation of how you have done elaborate things in the past in a vain attempt to lose weight.

Praise God! Verse 8 tells us that there is a better way. Who, according to Micah 6:8, is the One who shows us what is good?

What predictably happens when we turn to man-made solutions rather than listen to God's simple instructions, especially when it comes to the way we nourish and care for our wonderfully made-by-God bodies?

In verse 8, God, through the prophet Micah, asks, "What does the LORD require of you?" Micah immediately tells us three things our Lord wants us to do. What are those three things?

How are you acting justly when you follow the health and fitness guidelines that are part of the First Place 4 Health program? (Remember that treating yourself justly is as important to God as treating others fairly!)

We are next told "to love mercy." Recall from Day Two of our Week Two study that Jesus saved us because of His great mercy. How are we showing great mercy to ourselves and to others when we bring our lives into conformity with God's will and way when it comes to loving self-care?

Finally, we are asked "to walk humbly with our God." Reflecting on what you have learned in yesterday's lesson, how is daily prayer part of walking humbly with God?

When you mistreat the wonderfully made body that God created and called good, are you walking humbly with God? Why or why not?

How is following the principles of the First Place 4 Health program part of walking humbly with God?

What are you doing when you neglect any one part of the First Place 4 Health program, even though you religiously apply some of the other aspects of self-care?

When you give Christ first place in your life, what is your priority, and how is daily prayer part of the lifestyle that pleases God?

Thank You, loving Lord, for giving me simple but specific instructions so that I clearly understand what You require of me. Forgive me for those times in the past when I have done elaborate things rather than simply listening to Your Word and doing what it says. Amen.

Day 4

THE BENEFITS OF TRUSTING GOD

Gracious God, all wisdom comes from You. Today I pray that You will continue to teach me how to walk humbly with You, for You are my God and I desire to do what is pleasing to You. Amen.

Proverbs 3:5-8 contains timeless wisdom about another inner attitude that is pleasing to God—and will bring health to the body! For those of us who are intent on restoring the damage that years of negligent self-care have wrought on our physical bodies, this is indeed good news! So turn to those verses now, as we look at more of God's simple instructions.

Proverbs 3:5 is a command. The first part of the command reads:

__________ in the __________ with __________ your __________.

What is the importance of the word "all" in this command?

But in order to "trust in the LORD with all your heart," there is something you cannot continue to do. What must you stop doing?

And ______ not on ______ own ______.

How were the health and fitness measures you took prior to joining First Place 4 Health part of leaning on your own understanding? Give a thorough explanation!

What makes First Place 4 Health different, and how is this program part of trusting God with all your heart?

Proverbs 3:6 contains a wonderful promise. What does the Lord agree to do for us when we acknowledge Him in all our ways?

What does the presence of the word "all" in this verse reaffirm?

According to verse 7 of Proverbs 3, what two things are we to do instead of being wise in our own eyes?

When we trust in the Lord with all our heart and refuse to be wise in our own eyes, what happens (see Proverbs 3:8)?

Can we really expect to be restored to health and vitality when we insist on doing things our way rather than God's way? Reflect on what you learned in Proverbs 3:5-8, and thoroughly explain your answer.

How is daily prayer part of the trust in God that leads us on a straight path and restores us to health and wholeness?

How is not being wise in our own eyes part of surrendering our will and way to the Lordship of Jesus Christ?

O Lord God Almighty, I humbly confess that all too often I have ignored Your Word and run after what seemed wise in my own eyes. Please forgive me, Lord, for not listening to You and following the path You clearly set before me. Amen.

FAITH THAT PLEASES GOD

Day 5

O Lord, Your mercies are new every morning and Your faithfulness is great. Today I ask that You continue to show me the path that will lead to restoration and wholeness as I read and meditate on Your Word. Amen.

Hebrews 11 is a tribute to the men and women of faith who have gone before us. According to Romans 15:4, these courageous faith stories are included in God's Word for a very specific reason: "to teach us, so that through endurance and the encouragement of the Scriptures we might have hope." How is the inclusion of these stories in the Bible part of God's daily provision for our needs?

Sandwiched between the wonderful faith stories in Hebrews 11, we find another short verse that contains God's simple instructions for those who desire to please Him and put Him first in all things. Turn to Hebrews 11:6. No matter what else we may do, it is impossible to please God without one thing. According to Hebrews 11:6, what is that one thing?

Hebrews 11:6 goes on to tell us what faith looks like. When we come to God we must:

__________ that he __________ and that he __________ those who __________ __________ him.

Using the truth contained in Hebrews 11:6 as the basis for your answer, how is coming to God in prayer an act of faith?

If you did not believe that God exists, would you pray? If you did not believe God rewards those who earnestly seek Him, would you seek Him? Prayer is an act of faith, a way of pleasing God.

Our memory verse for this week tells us an amazing thing about the reward of seeking God in prayer. Write the verse below, and then underline the benefit we receive when we come to God in prayer.

The phrase "whatever you ask for" in that verse can be deceptive unless we consider it in light of the other teachings in the Bible. We can never base our faith on one isolated verse, pulled out of context. When we erroneously rely on one verse rather the whole counsel of God, we set ourselves up for disappointment and failure. And so it is with this week's memory verse. As you think about the words of this week's memory verse, stop and ask yourself, *Would a loving God give me something that would ultimately be harmful to me, even though in my own eyes it is very desirable?* Explain your answer, based on what you have learned so far in the *Begin with Christ* Bible study.

What would happen if you were to ask for something that was contrary to God's will and way? Would God still answer that prayer and give you what was right in your own eyes, even though He would have to violate His own principles to do so? Why or why not?

Hebrews 11:6 tells us that in order to please God, we must "earnestly seek him." Is praying for something that is contrary to God's revealed will earnestly seeking Him? Explain your answer.

Is praying for something outside of God's will an act of faith or an act of foolishness? Give your answer careful thought before writing it down.

We know that it is God's will that we have a healthy and fit body, a clear mind, balanced emotions and a well-nourished spirit. How is praying daily for success in your First Place 4 Health efforts a prayer that your God will honor because you are earnestly seeking to do the things that you know please Him?

After you pray for success in First Place 4 Health, what do you then need to do?

O Lord, I know that in order to please You, I must believe that You exist and that You will reward me when I earnestly seek You. Thank You for hearing my prayer and accepting my words as an act of faith. Amen.

Day 6

REFLECTION AND APPLICATION

O Lord, please teach me to pray! Amen.

This week our *Begin with Christ* Bible study lesson has been about building spiritual strength, stability and stamina through the daily discipline of prayer. But prayer is not something we can learn just by reading words, any more than we can learn to do a physical exercise just by reading the how-to instructions in a book. In order to get the full benefit of this week's teaching on prayer, we must put into action what we have learned.

To really learn about prayer, we must pray! Unfortunately, many of us have a faulty perception about the words we must use when we talk to God. Too often when we think about praying, the first thing that comes to mind are images of people praying lofty prayers in church—prayers full of "Thees" and "Thous," and words that most of us don't even understand. But true prayer is a conversation with God, talking to Him much like we would talk to a trusted counselor or friend, not using high and lofty language. Yes, God is to be reverenced and His name is to be respected, but that does not mean we must learn a new language to speak to our Father in heaven. God's universal language, His native tongue, is the language of a loving heart.

When we first begin the daily discipline of prayer, writing our prayers helps us focus our words and thoughts as we talk to our Father in heaven. So today, rather than reading words about prayer, we are going to actually pray!

Your assignment is to write a prayer to God, much like you would write a letter (or an email) to a dear friend who is away on an extended journey. Your spiritual journal is an ideal place to record this prayer-letter. Write from your heart, and tell God about your hopes and dreams, your fears and anxieties, as you begin this lifelong journey to restoration and renewed health. Begin your prayer by thanking God for listening to you, and end your prayer with thanksgiving because you are confident that God will answer your prayer in His will, His way and His perfect timing. The only wrong way to do this exercise is to not do it at all, so begin your conversation with God now.

Thank You, Father, that I can come to You in prayer, confident that You hear my words and will put spiritual forces in motion to bring an answer, even as my words are being written on the page before me. Amen.

REFLECTION AND APPLICATION

O gracious and loving God, help me to live and move and have my being in You so that my whole life becomes an act of prayer. Amen.

All too often we think of prayer as a passive activity, something we do while seated in our comfortable quiet-time chair or kneeling beside our bed. But as we read through the pages of Scripture, we find that prayer was often combined with physical movement—dancing, singing, marching into battle. So today, rather than sitting and writing out our prayers, we are going to lace up our tennis shoes and opt for prayer in motion. You can choose whatever type of movement you want to combine with your prayer, but make it an activity you enjoy. Prayer in motion is a way of expressing your gratitude to God for the marvelous things He has done for you. It should never be an endurance contest! This is your opportunity to show your thankfulness by moving the wonderfully made body God created to be sleek and agile.

Just as with yesterday's written prayer assignment, the only wrong way to do this prayer exercise is to not do it at all! Don't be concerned about looking foolish in your own eyes or in the eyes of others. Your Father in heaven takes great delight when His children praise Him with their bodies, because it honors His wonderfully made, carefully handcrafted creation. Today is the day to pick up your feet, swing your arms, sway your body and lift your voice in prayer to the God of all creation!

Group Prayer Requests

first place 4 health

Today's Date: ____________________

Name	Request

Results

____

____

____

____

____

____

____

Week Four

joyful obedience is the pathway to blessing

SCRIPTURE MEMORY VERSE

Whoever has my commands and obeys them, he is the one who loves me. He who loves me will be loved by my Father, and I too will love him and show myself to him.

JOHN 14:21

If beginning with Christ just entailed getting to know Jesus—the One who has supremacy in all things—and spending time in pleasant conversation with Him, then our success in First Place 4 Health would be guaranteed! Yes, it is exciting to learn about Jesus, to watch Him minister to the downtrodden and despairing. We delight as we see Him restore health and wholeness and bring peace and joy to those who are weary and oppressed. The more we learn about this man called Jesus the Christ, the more we are convinced that He does deserve first place in all areas of our life. Talking to God in prayer becomes our joy and delight. What at first seemed awkward quickly gives way to warm, intimate conversation—soon quiet time with our Lord is a sacred spot in our day that we look forward to with eager anticipation.

But an ongoing relationship with Jesus Christ requires more than just knowing our Lord and spending time talking to Him. In the weeks ahead, we will focus on other aspects of our relationship with God, some that will be pleasant and easy to apply and others that will be difficult and may incite our resistance. At each juncture on our journey to success, we have a choice that determines whether we will move forward or fall back. Each time we are asked to put a new behavior into practice, we can either surrender to God's life-giving will and way, or we can resist, rebel and turn back to our old self-destructive ways. We can either move on to the next lesson, or we can stay stuck in the past—and the choice is ours to make. The God who gave us free will does not impose Himself or His purposes on us. We get to make the choice; we get to reap the consequences, either good or bad.

This week's *Begin with Christ* lessons are pivotal points where falling back may seem easier than moving forward. Left to our own devices, we will balk at this point. It is one thing to know Jesus and to spend time talking to Him. It is quite another to obey Him—not just begrudgingly obey Him in outward things while our heart is far from Him, but joyfully obey Him with all our heart, mind, spirit and strength. Like it or not, joyful obedience is the only pathway to blessing. As our Scripture memory verse for the week reminds us, those who love Jesus keep His commands.

Day 1

THROW OFF THE THINGS THAT HINDER

O loving and gracious Lord, open my eyes so that I can see the truth of Your Word; and once I have seen the truth, give me the ability to courageously obey, always looking to Jesus, the author and finisher of my faith. Amen.

In the physical world, our daily workout includes such things as walking, running, swimming and working out with weights—things that require specific physical movements. All too often we are prone to think of spiritual exercise as more passive—that it includes such things as reading, journaling and quietly praying. However, the Word of God tells us a different story. We are instructed to cast off our cares (see 1 Peter 5:7), put on the full armor of God (see Ephesians 6:13-17), run with perseverance and throw off the things that hinder us (see Hebrews 12:1), and dance and make music (see Psalm 149:3). Hardly passive endeavors!

Last week our Bible study took us to Hebrews 11, and this week we are going to look at Hebrews 12. Turn to Hebrews 12:1 in your Bible, and begin today's lesson by prayerfully reading this verse.

The unknown writer of the book of Hebrews begins chapter 12 by looking back at the giants of the faith described in chapter 11. What does the writer of Hebrews call those who have gone before us?

Stop for a moment and consider the implications of those words! You have "a great cloud of witnesses"! How will knowing that fact impact your behavior the next time you are tempted to fall back into old, destructive habits? Explain your answer.

And because we have that great cloud of witnesses, there are two specific actions we are exhorted to do:

Let us ______ ______ everything that ______ and the ______ that so easily entangles, and let us ______ with perseverance the ______ marked out before us.

As you contemplate the things that hinder you and the sins that entangle you, be mindful of the fact that the things that hinder you are usually external circumstances, while the sins that entangle you are within. Identify one thing that hinders you in regard to your First Place 4 Health efforts.

What do you need to do today to be obedient to the command to throw off that hindrance? It could be something like eliminating the junk food in your kitchen cabinets, rearranging your schedule so that you have time to exercise or getting up early so that you can spend quiet time with God. Make your answer specific to your situation.

How might throwing off what hinders you be like casting your cares on God because He cares for you? (You might want to look back at Day Two of our Week Three study.)

For our purposes in First Place 4 Health, the course marked out for us is giving Christ first place in caring for our mind, heart, body and spirit. With regard to your First Place 4 Health program, what is the sin that easily entangles you and keeps you from running the race marked out for you? Think of one very specific behavior that continues to trip you up in spite of your good intentions.

What specific step or steps can you take today to throw off that sinful behavior so that you can run the race marked out for you?

Throwing off the things that hinder us and the sins that easily entangle us is one of the choice points we spoke about in the introduction to this week's Bible study. Are you going to do what it takes to throw off these obstacles, or are you going to fall back into old destructive patterns of behavior? Explain both your answer and the specific steps you will take to be obedient as a reflection of your love for Jesus and of His love for you.

O loving Lord, You have given me everything I need to live a life that pleases You, even a great cloud of witnesses. Thank You for Jesus, the author and finisher of my faith, the One I can follow with confidence. Amen.

Day 2

OBEDIENCE PERSEVERES

O Lord, I pray You will give me knowledge and good judgment so that I can run with perseverance the race set before me. Amen.

During yesterday's lesson, we looked at the importance of throwing off all the things that hinder and entangle us and keep us from running the race marked out before us. But there is one word we did not talk about as we looked at this specific aspect of obedience, and that word is "perseverance." Open your Bible and reread Hebrews 12:1, making note of the placement of the word "perseverance." Why do you think the writer of Hebrews used the words "with perseverance" to describe the race we are to run?

Look up "perseverance" in a dictionary. What does the word mean? Write the definition below.

What words in the definition especially spoke to you with regard to your efforts to throw off the things that hinder you?

In the words of a popular saying, we might say that perseverance means "keepin' on keepin' on." What does perseverance tell us about obedience? Is it a one-time choice or an ongoing decision to do everything our Lord asks us to do? Explain your answer.

How does the word "perseverance" help you understand the importance of choosing a health and fitness program that you can follow for a lifetime? In giving your answer, remember that we are either moving forward or we are falling back. In the battle against the things that entangle us and drag us down, there is no neutral ground.

Through the words of the apostle John in Revelation 2, the risen Christ sent a message to the saints in the church at Ephesus. In verse 2 of this message, the living Lord commended them for three things:

I know your ______________, your ______________ ______________ and your ______________.

How do these three things work together, and what would happen to the first two if perseverance were missing?

If the risen Lord were speaking to you about your First Place 4 Health efforts, could He commend you for your deeds, hard work and perseverance? Why or why not?

Now look at Revelation 2:7. What blessing is promised for those who hear the Lord's words and overcome the things that hinder them?

Based on what you have learned thus far in the *Begin with Christ* Bible study, what is the pathway to receiving this blessing?

O sovereign Lord, obeying You one time is easy; perseverance is not. Please give me the grace to endure the course You have marked out before me in First Place 4 Health. Amen.

Day 3

FOLLOW THE LEADER

Gracious Lord, You have given me everything I need, including a leader I can look to and follow. Thank You for Jesus, who came to Earth in human flesh to show me the way. Amen.

Unlike some authority figures who ask that we do as they say but not as they do, Jesus never asks His disciples to do anything He was not first willing to do Himself. This is especially true when it comes to obedience. According to Hebrews 12:2, Jesus is "the author and perfecter of our faith" because He came to Earth in human form so that we could follow His lead and learn from Him how to obey God. Today we will continue our studies in Hebrews 12, so open your Bible and read verses 1-3, recalling what you have already learned from our study of verse 1.

After exhorting us to run with perseverance the race set before us by throwing off everything that hinders and entangles us, the writer of Hebrews tells us to follow the leader, the One who has gone before us to show us the way. What is the action step we are told to take in Hebrews 12:2?

What does "fix our eyes on Jesus" mean? Describe the visual image conjured up for you by that phrase.

If your eyes are fixed on Jesus, what are you not looking at?

What visual temptations do you face in your everyday environment? Think about the things your eyes fix themselves on, things that trip you up and hinder you from running the race set before you in First Place 4 Health. We live in a visual society that entices us in many ways, so be creative as you think of the places your eyes gaze when they are not fixed on Jesus. (Bear in mind that there is a difference between "seeing" and "fixing our eyes"!)

The writer of Hebrews goes on in verse 2 to describe Jesus. How is Jesus "the author and perfecter" of your faith when it comes to participation in the First Place 4 Health program? (It might help you to think of the "author" as the one who writes the script and the "perfecter" as the director who shows you how to play your assigned role so that your actions conform to the author's design.)

How does the fact that Jesus is both author and perfecter of your faith journey in First Place 4 Health give you hope and encouragement?

With Jesus as the author and perfecter of your faith, what is your part?

Are you running the First Place 4 Health course with your eyes fixed on Jesus and your ears attuned to the encouragement you are receiving as you read the faith stories of those who form the great cloud of witnesses? Why or why not?

How are both Jesus and the great cloud of witnesses part of God's ongoing provision for your daily needs? Make your answer relative to your participation in First Place 4 Health.

Gracious and loving Lord, thank You for going before me to show me the way to run with perseverance the course marked out before me. I know I can only run the good race because You are the author and the perfecter of my faith, the One who sets the course and steadies my feeble steps. Amen.

JOYFUL OBEDIENCE

Day 4

O loving Lord, thank You for coming to Earth in human form to show me how to run with joy the race set before me. Amen.

Jesus is indeed the author and the perfecter of our faith, the One who marks out our course and steadies our steps, the One who has gone before us to show us the way. How does this truth correspond to one of the "I Am" statements that you learned about during Day Four of our Week Two study? (Either turn to that day's study, or look at John 14:6 for the answer.)

Jesus not only ran the course set before Him by His Father in heaven but also ran the race for a reason. Turn back to Hebrews 12:2 in your Bible. We are told:

Jesus . . . for the ________ set before him ________ the ________, ________ its ________.

According to the last part of Hebrews 12:2, why was Jesus willing to suffer—what was the joy Jesus looked forward to?

In taking His place at the right hand of the throne of God, Jesus' work here on Earth was complete. He entered into His Father's joy and took His seat at God's right hand. His earthly work was finished. He had indeed run the race and honorably completed the course. He had been victorious!

What is the joy you look forward to as you run the First Place 4 Health course set out before you? Since we are not just focusing our efforts on one aspect of our being, list a joy set before you for each aspect of your being.

Physically: ______________________________

____

Mentally: ______________________________

____

Emotionally: ______________________________

____

Spiritually: ______________________________

____

Before He could experience the joy He looked forward to, Jesus "endured the cross, scorning its shame." Rewrite those words to describe what you will need to endure in order to experience the joy set before you in the First Place 4 Health program.

____

____

____

____

What would have happened if Jesus had opted for immediate gratification instead of patient perseverance when He faced the painful ordeal before Him?

____

____

____

____

What will happen if you opt for immediate gratification rather than go through the painful ordeal of throwing off all the things that hinder you so that you can run with perseverance?

In terms of your First Place 4 Health program, what might immediate gratification look like? Your answer should include the people, places or things that give you on-the-spot pleasure but sabotage your long-term goals.

Does your answer to the previous question bear any resemblance to the things that hinder and the sins that entangle that we looked at earlier this week? Why or why not?

What lesson did you learn from Jesus, the author and perfecter of your faith, as you completed today's lesson?

Sovereign Lord, so often I look at the pleasure of the moment rather than fix my eyes on Jesus and follow His lead. Forgive me for not seeing the joy You have set before me and then making that joy my focus and my goal. Amen.

Day 5

OPPOSITION

Lord God, help me to be patient and kind to those who oppose my First Place 4 Health efforts. Following Jesus' example, I will entrust myself to You and continue to do good. Amen.

It would be difficult enough to overcome the things that hinder us and the sins that easily entangle us if we lived our lives in isolation! However, most of us must continue to interact with others as we undertake this process of restoring our lives to health, wholeness and balance. Going off into the desert or staying in a mountaintop retreat, as desirable as either one of those things might seem, just isn't an option for us! We must continue to live and move and have our being in a world full of temptation and opposition. We are called to be in the world.

During this week's study, we have seen the importance of fixing our eyes on Jesus, the author and perfecter of our faith. Today we will continue to look to Jesus and follow His example, as found in Hebrews 12:1-3. Read those verses now, and recall the lessons you have already learned from Jesus in our study of verses 1 and 2.

Verse 3 begins with another action command. What is the first word of Hebrews 12:3?

According to Hebrews 12:3, who is it we are to consider?

What did the One we are to consider do?

Who were the ones who opposed Jesus?

Why are we to "consider him who endured such opposition from sinful men"?

How is not growing weary and losing heart related to the perseverance we learned about in our Day Two study?

It is easy to understand why Jesus was opposed by sinful men, those who wanted to thwart His efforts and undermine His purpose. However, being able to apply that concept to our First Place 4 Health efforts is a bit more difficult—but every bit as necessary! Jesus is our example so that *we* will not grow weary and lose heart. We know that Jesus endured opposition. What does that truth tell us that we should also be prepared to face?

Who might oppose your efforts in First Place 4 Health, and why might they oppose you? Remember that others close to you, others who are not motivated to change, will be impacted by your new lifestyle and behavior. Eating healthy meals and exercising is not what they want to do right now! Others may oppose you because to admit you were right would convict them of their own need to change. Some may be envious, secretly wanting a healthy, balanced lifestyle, but not being willing to do the hard work. Perhaps those close to you are afraid you will not care about them, or you will not continue to meet their needs, because of your participation in First Place 4 Health. Instead of encouraging you, they might try to discourage you. Not all the people who oppose you are sinful, of course, but some are. Think of the way people and companies who are more concerned with monetary profit than your health and well-being might oppose your First Place 4 Health efforts. Think carefully before you describe your opposition.

How can all this opposition—some subtle and some blatant—cause you to become weary and lose heart?

What did Jesus, our example, do when He encountered opposition (see Hebrews 12:3)?

Consider him who ____________ such opposition.

Part of running with endurance the race set before you is anticipating opposition. Consider how you might be able to endure the opposition you will encounter in the days, weeks, months and years ahead. Unless you come up with an action plan, you will quickly fall prey to those who oppose you, so be thorough in your answer!

O merciful Lord, You do provide all I need to live a life of holiness. Thank You for Jesus, who has gone before me to show me how to endure opposition. By the power of Your Holy Spirit, please continue to guide me into all truth so that I can run the race before me with endurance. Amen.

REFLECTION AND APPLICATION

Day 6

Thank You for giving me everything I need, precious Lord, even the ability to recognize the people, places and things that have the ability to throw me off course and thwart my First Place 4 Health goals. Amen.

During our Bible study time yesterday, we looked at some very difficult questions—questions that asked us to consider how we will handle those who will oppose our First Place 4 Health efforts. A universal kingdom-of-God truth that we often forget is that temptation always follows commitment, and that principle will certainly prove itself true once you have made a commitment to a balanced, healthy lifestyle!

Throughout salvation history, we see this pattern repeat itself over and over again. Whenever someone makes a commitment to serve God, the evil one is always lurking in the shadows, ready to offer temptation and transform that commitment into failure. Even Jesus, immediately following His baptism, was taken to the desert wilderness to be tempted.

As Christ followers, we can learn to anticipate this pattern. And anticipating this pattern, we can prepare ourselves for what lies ahead. Just as soon as we make a commitment to spiritual growth and change, we will suddenly become aware of just how much temptation there is in our everyday environment. People, places and things that test our resolve and dampen our desire to persevere bombard us from every direction. It is so easy to fall back into old, destructive habits and patterns of behavior; the evil one is always close at hand, doing all he can do to throw us off course.

Temptation in the wake of commitment is why the spiritual dimension of First Place 4 Health is essential to being able to run with perseverance the race set before us. Through the spiritual discipline of Bible study, Scripture reading, prayer, Scripture memory work and encouraging others, we draw from a power inside us that is greater than the temptation that surrounds us (see 1 John 4:4). Although most of us come into First Place 4 Health because we want to lose weight, the moment we make First Place 4 Health just about what we eat, we have set ourselves up to fail.

In addition to mental resolve, we need divine weapons to ward off the attacks of the evil one, our archenemy who waits on the sidelines, ready to lure us into temptation. First Place 4 Health is about balance. And part of that balance is utilizing the power within us to overcome the strongholds we are powerless to overcome on our own. Joyful obedience requires that we be continually mindful of the commitment-temptation cycle. Awareness allows us to protect ourselves with the whole armor of God so that we can stand firm in His mighty power and resist the wiles of the devil.

During yesterday's study, you were asked to compile a list of those who might oppose your First Place 4 Health efforts. You were also asked to come up with a plan so that you would be able to gracefully handle that opposition without falling prey to the temptation to grow weary and lose heart. If you have not completed those lists, spend more time with them today. It is essential that you identify those who have the potential to sabotage your First Place 4 Health program. That knowledge will allow you to come up with a perseverance plan before you find yourself falling back into old behaviors because the pain of opposition is more immediate than the joy of obedience through delayed gratification.

O Lord, You are my strength and my shield, the One who gives me the courage to stand up to those who oppose me because my eyes are fixed on Jesus and I am following His example. Amen.

Day 7

REFLECTION AND APPLICATION

Sovereign Lord, often I wish I could just go away to a quiet place and spend my time with You. But You have called me to be a witness to Your goodness and grace, even in the midst of this transition process. Please give me the grace to proclaim Your goodness in all that I say and do. Amen.

Fire swept through one end of a local strip mall, destroying several shops. The other stores in the mall, although not damaged by the fire itself, suffered smoke damage and the water used to extinguish the fire doused neighboring shops, too. In the wake of the disaster, the strip-mall owner decided to remodel the entire center. However, many of the shop owners could not afford to close during the remodeling process, so most stores stayed open for business. A banner in front of the shops announced "Open During Remodeling," while another sign cautioned "Please Watch Your Step." As hesitant shoppers walked through the temporary entrance, they passed a pile of rubble and debris on their right and a stack of building materials on their left.

For many of us in First Place 4 Health, this scene is an analogy of our life. We, too, have been damaged and need to be remodeled, but just like these merchants, we must stay open for business. We cannot shut the doors of our life during the remodeling process. Unlike those merchants, however, we can't hang a sign around our neck that reads "Open During Remodeling, but Please Watch Your Step."

Yes, we are First Place 4 Health members who desperately need remodeling—but we still need to be spouses, parents, friends and workers as we journey toward wholeness and health. Even though we can't retreat to a private place while the Holy Spirit rebuilds our disheveled lives, we *can* realize we are under construction, and we can vow to take good care of ourselves during the remodeling process, even in the face of opposition. We can get plenty of rest when the old debris is on one side and the new material has not yet been put into place. Spending time each day in God's Word will help us keep our balance and establish healthy habits that will be part of the newly remodeled creation Christ is bringing forth. We can share our need for more solitude with our family and close friends, asking that they support our need for more time with our Lord.

Our First Place 4 Health group can be compassionate encouragers who are also wearing invisible "Open During Remodeling" signs. "Endurance" means being patient during the process, always remembering that Jesus is the author and the perfecter of our faith. He will bring to completion the good work He has begun. No matter how difficult the course may seem, we can endure because we know that God isn't finished with us yet!

My Lord and my God, today I give You thanks and praise, even though I am in the midst of a major remodeling process and am often overwhelmed by the work that lies before me. Yet I can rejoice in the middle of the mess because I am confident that You will complete the good work You have begun in me. You will never leave me or desert me. You have promised to be my leader, my guide and my companion on this track to health, wholeness and balance that honors You. Amen.

Group Prayer Requests

first place 4 health

Today's Date: ____________________

Name	Request

Results

____

____

____

____

____

____

____

Week Five

our folly and God's forgiveness

SCRIPTURE MEMORY VERSE

You know my folly, O God;
my guilt is not hidden from you.

PSALM 69:5

Sin is not a popular subject in our society. People try to soft-soap sin and call it by other names. They try to minimize and ignore it, and often they even try to call what is evil good and what is good evil. But God is not fooled by our excuses or by our fancy words. In His kingdom, sin is an affront to a just and holy God, a God who calls His people to be separate and set apart, to be holy because He is holy. Rather than trying to hide or disguise our sin, we are asked by our merciful and compassionate Father to come to Him and confess our sins, not so that He can punish us, but so that He can forgive us. Trying to whitewash our sins only increases our guilt. But the moment we confess our sins, God is faithful to "forgive us our sins and purify us from all unrighteousness" (1 John 1:9). That is the good news of the Gospel of Jesus Christ. In Christ, God is no longer counting our sins against us. Jesus, the One who had done no wrong, took everything that we had ever done wrong and paid the penalty on our behalf. He took on all of our sins; we received all of His righteousness. Amazing grace!

For those of us who are seeking to restore the years our folly and out-of-control living have taken away, forgiveness plays an important role, because forgiveness is an essential part of our recovery. Only when God forgives our sins are we free to choose the path that leads to health, restoration and wholeness. Until our sins are forgiven, we are doomed to repeat the mistakes of our past, much like a moth is drawn to a flame. Confession clears the path ahead of us and erases the sins behind us. After the psalmist David had been forgiven of the sins that he had committed against God, he declared, "Blessed are those whose transgressions are forgiven, whose sins are covered. Blessed are those whose sin the LORD does not count against them and in whose spirit is no deceit" (Psalm 32:1-2, *TNIV*). That same blessing can be ours when we are willing to confess our sins and accept God's unconditional forgiveness.

Day 1

IN THE BEGINNING

O Lord, You teach me what is right and lead me along straight paths. Today I pray You will send the Holy Spirit to expose my folly so that I can come to You and receive forgiveness. Amen.

In the beginning, God created Adam and Eve and placed them in a beautiful garden. But Adam and Eve were not content with the good things God had given them; they wanted the one thing God had told them was forbidden—and, of course, it had to do with food! Turn to Genesis 3:1-3 in your Bible as we begin to learn about what happened that fateful day.

Four people were in the garden that morning. Who were they? (Hint: The serpent is identified in Revelation 12:9 as Satan, the one who tries to lead the whole world astray. The fourth person is implied but not specifically mentioned.)

How did the serpent, true to his purpose, lead Eve astray?

How does your ancient foe lead you astray with questions that cause you to doubt God's love and mercy, especially as it applies to being deprived of foods that you would like to be able to eat but that are outside the Live It plan?

Answering the serpent was Eve's second mistake. What was her first?

When we listen to the crafty voice of temptation instead of immediately destroying every word that is contrary to the Word of God, we have made our first mistake! The minute we try to formulate an answer, we are flirting with sin. How like the serpent's voice are commercials and other advertisements that encourage you to eat food that is not part of your Live It plan?

When Eve answered the serpent, she made yet another mistake. Read Eve's words in Genesis 3:3, and then contrast them with God's words in Genesis 2:17. What is different?

What happens to us when we try to change God's words to suit our purposes or to win a debate rather than just quoting exactly what God has said?

Think of a recent time when Satan appeared to you with a question that caused you to doubt God's love and mercy, and then trace how things went downhill from there. As you have done elsewhere in this study, make your answer relevant to health and fitness.

How is Scripture memory an important part of repelling the temptations of the evil one, lest we, like Eve, fall into sin?

Compassionate God, how it must break Your Father's heart when You see me flirting with sin. Forgive me, Lord, for not listening to every word You say and then following Your simple instructions. Amen.

Day 2

BE CAREFUL, LITTLE EYES

Gracious God, You tell me to fix my eyes on Jesus, the author and perfecter of my faith, but all too often my eyes end up fixed on the cause of my undoing. Please forgive me. Today I pray that You will help me see the truth so that the truth can set me free. Amen.

In Sunday School, many of us learned a song called "Oh, Be Careful Little Eyes." If you know that song, you might want to sing the parts you can remember before we begin today's lesson!

Today we are going to resume our study of folly and forgiveness back in the beginning, this time picking up where we left off yesterday. Turn to Genesis 3 and read verses 1-7. As you read verses 1-3, recall what you learned in yesterday's lesson.

How many times do you see the words "eyes," "eye" and "saw" in verses 4-7?

____

____

____

Verse 6 tells us:

The woman __________ that the fruit of the tree was good for food and pleasing to the __________.

How do you think that Eve could tell by looking at the fruit that it was good for food?

____

____

____

Do you think the fact that the food was "pleasing to the eye" had something to do with her choice to eat the fruit? In answering this question, recall the last time you saw a decadent dessert on a magazine cover or a grocery-store display.

Which was more appealing to you: the nutritional content of the food or the appearance?

Now read 1 John 2:15-17 in your Bible. We will be studying these verses in depth later in our *Begin with Christ* Bible study, but for now let's concentrate on the role our eyes play in leading us into sin. In this verse, John talks about the lust of sinful people's eyes. How does the lust of your eyes lead you into sin, just like it led to the downfall of our first parents, Adam and Eve? Be specific in your answer.

How is protecting your eyes part of the health and balance of the First Place 4 Health program, and how might visual stimulation be part of the list of things that hinder you?

How can you protect yourself from falling into temptation because of what your eyes see? Be creative in your solutions to the "lust of the eyes" problem.

When Christ is first in your life, what is your focus and priority?

O Lord, how foolish I must look to You when I let the things my eyes see lead me into sin. Help me to keep my eyes on Jesus and not be lured into the temptations that surround me in this world. Amen.

Day 3 GOD SEES, TOO!

O Lord, You know my folly, and my guilt is not hidden from You. Forgive me when I try to hide rather than run toward You to receive Your mercy and grace. Amen.

Although God does not have physical eyes like we do, the Bible is very clear that God can see! As a matter of fact, 2 Chronicles 16:9 contains an awesome promise for those who are seeking to put Christ first in all things: "For the eyes of the LORD range throughout the earth to strengthen those whose hearts are fully committed to Him." Pause for a moment and thank God for strengthening you when His ever-present eyes see that your heart is fully committed to keeping Christ first in all things.

God's eyes don't just range throughout the earth to strengthen His faithful people. What else does our memory verse for this week tell us God's eyes see? Write out the memory verse and underline the parts of that verse that answer this question.

During our Day One study this week, we learned that there were four people in the garden the day Adam and Eve fell into sin. Adam was there, Eve was there and Satan, in the guise of a serpent, was there. Who else was there?

Let's resume our study of Genesis 3 by turning to verses 8-13. Carefully read this part of the story. Verse 8 tells us that Adam and Eve heard something. What did they hear?

What did Adam and Eve do when they heard the Lord walking in the garden?

Verse 9 tells us that God called out to Adam, asking a question. What was the question God asked?

Did God ask Adam the question because He didn't know where Adam and Eve were hiding? And if not, why do you think God asked the question?

What was Adam's answer?

What does our memory verse tell us about trying to hide from God?

Recall a time when you wanted to hide from God because you felt naked and exposed and were afraid of the consequences of your behavior.

In Genesis 3:11, God replied to Adam's confession by asking two more questions. Read those questions carefully. Who told Adam he was naked? Was it God, Satan or Adam's own conscience?

When you have eaten something that is not on your Live It plan (or have failed to exercise or do the other things on your daily First Place 4 Health routine), do you need anyone to remind you that you have not been faithful to God's plan for your life? Why or why not?

Rather than just confess that he had sinned, Adam did something else—he used what is commonly called "The Genesis 3:12 Defense." Exactly what did Adam do?

In like fashion, Eve used The Genesis 3:12 Defense, too. Who did Eve blame?

When was the last time you used The Genesis 3:12 Defense to excuse your folly, especially as it applied to eating food that did not promote health and wholeness? And whom did you blame?

Is God fooled by The Genesis 3:12 Defense, or is it part of the folly we are seeking to hide? Explain your answer.

Even though Adam and Eve had disobeyed God, God made provision to cover their nakedness. Genesis 3:7 tells us that Adam and Eve tried to cover their nakedness by sewing fig leaves together, much the way we try to cover up our sin rather than confess it to God. Turn to Genesis 3:21. What did God do to cover Adam's and Eve's nakedness?

In order to cover Adam and Eve with garments of skin, what did God have to do?

What was that first animal sacrifice symbolic of? (If you aren't sure of the answer, read Hebrews 9:28.)

Spend the rest of your quiet time today thanking God that your sins are covered by the precious blood of Jesus Christ, the Lamb of God whose blood covers all your unrighteousness.

O Lord, please forgive me for the times I try to cover up my sin or attempt to blame others rather than coming to You in heartfelt sorrow and repentance. Amen.

YOU CAN RUN, BUT YOU CAN'T HIDE

Day 4

All-knowing, all-seeing God, You know me better than I know myself, and You love me anyway. Thank You for accepting me where I am and loving me too much to leave me here. Help me to rejoice in Your presence, today, tomorrow and always. Amen.

Throughout salvation history, people have tried to run rather than listen to God's voice—and obey His words. Adam and Eve were first, and there have been many who have followed in their footsteps. King David, the great king of Israel, the "man after [God's] own heart," learned the hard way that he could not hide his sin from God (1 Samuel 13:14). Like Eve, David took his eyes off God and fell into sin—in David's case, the sin of adultery, after he saw a beautiful woman bathing. After a long chain of events in which one sin led to another, David took Bathsheba into his palace as if he had done nothing wrong. But 2 Samuel 11 ends with a sobering truth: "The thing David had done displeased the Lord" (verse 27). Later, after David had confessed his sin, he wrote Psalm 32, which speaks about the blessings of forgiveness. David wrote this week's memory verse, as well as another psalm to teach others the futility of trying to hide from God.

Turn to Psalm 139 in your Bible, and read verses 1-12. What is the first thing you notice as you read this psalm?

If David had realized he could not hide from God on that evening when he saw Bathsheba bathing, do you think he would have still fallen into sin? Why or why not?

What about Eve? Had she realized that God was in the garden that day, watching her as she flirted with temptation, do you think she would have eaten the forbidden fruit? Explain your answer.

And what about you? If you were always cognizant that God knows you better than you know yourself, would you still do things to damage the wonderfully made body He fashioned for you? Why or why not?

How does Psalm 139:1-12 affirm the words of our Scripture memory verse for the week? Write down this week's memory verse, and then note the parts of this verse that were repeated in Psalm 139:1-12.

In Psalm 139:5-6, David declared that the Lord hems him in "behind and before." Do you think David felt confined by God's perpetual presence or do you think it brought Him comfort?

What about you? Does the fact that God hems you in behind and before—that He knows what you are going to do before you even do it—make you feel confined, or is God's all-knowing presence a comfort to you? Why?

David ends Psalm 139 with a wonderful prayer we should daily make our own, and we will use it for our closing prayer today. After you have repeated these words, continue your prayer time by talking to God about how His perpetual presence brings you joy and delight.

> *Search me, O God, and know my heart; test me and know my anxious thoughts. See if there is any offensive way in me, and lead me in the way everlasting. Amen* (Psalm 139:23-24).

Day 5

FORGIVENESS GUARANTEED

Thank You, loving Lord, that You have called me to walk in the light. Today I pray that You will illuminate my mind so that I can benefit from Your teaching as I study Your Word. Amen.

During our studies this week, we have seen the folly of three of God's people, people who were intent on doing things their own way rather than surrendering to God's will and way. Recall how in all three examples, God's people allowed their eyes to lead them into sin. If we were to try to make a list of all those throughout the ages who have rebelled against God, there would not be enough room in even the largest of libraries to hold all the volumes that human folly would occupy. Fortunately, even though God's people continue to sin, God provided a once-and-for-all sacrifice to take away their guilt and shame. That once-and-for-all sacrifice was God's only Son, Jesus, who came to Earth in human form to save His people from their sins. The apostle John has some wonderful words for those who are in Christ Jesus. Turn to 1 John 1 in your Bible, and read verses 5-10.

John begins 1 John 1:5 by telling us where the message he is relaying came from. Who was the originator of this teaching? (You can look at 1 John 1:3 if you aren't sure of the correct answer.)

According to 1 John 1:5, "God is light." But He's not just a little light or a spotty light. How does John describe God's light?

As those called to walk in the light, what happens if we claim to have fellowship with Him yet continue to walk in the darkness (see 1 John 1:6)?

How is claiming to be part of the First Place 4 Health fellowship but continuing to live an out-of-control life akin to what John is describing in verse 6?

Conversely, what happens when we walk in the light and try to live by the truth? First John 1:7 gives us an awesome promise that has two benefits. What are those benefits?

Walking in the light provides us with fellowship; and Jesus' blood, the sacrifice of God's Son, purifies us from all of our sins! Pause for a moment and let that truth sink into your being!

Apparently in John's day, however—just as in ours—there were those who said they had not sinned. They were in denial! What do 1 John 1:8 and 10 teach us about saying we are without sin?

But praise God! Something wonderful happens when we confess our sins! First John 1:9 reads:

> If we ________ our ________, he is ________ and ________ and will ________ us our ________ and purify us from all unrighteousness.

When we try to hide our sins, we do not fool God, but we do cheat ourselves out of some marvelous benefits. Yet, as in all things, the choice is always ours to make. Which do you choose to do today, and why?

O compassionate Father, thank You for sending Jesus to die for my sins. Forgive me, Lord, for both the sins I commit and for the times I foolishly try to hide my folly from You. Amen.

Day 6

REFLECTION AND APPLICATION

Sovereign Lord, it is one thing to read about the folly of others but quite another to admit my own shortcomings. Please help me to tell myself the truth in love as I do this exercise today. Amen.

This week we looked at the folly of Adam and Eve, our first parents, and of King David, the great ruler of Israel. But confessing someone else's sins does not make us right with God! So today it is time to write our own folly story.

Think about a situation when your eyes led you into a temptation that resulted in sin. Maybe it was a trip to the grocery store, where some of the delicacies in the pastry aisle managed to jump right into your grocery cart and then went nonstop into your stomach! Or perhaps you bought that magazine to read about the latest diet craze and ended up making the aptly named Devilishly Sinful Chocolate Cake pictured on the cover instead. And then think about what you did in a vain attempt to cover up the weight you gained as a result of that folly.

Some folks binge and purge to try to avoid the consequences of overeating. Other's just purchase bigger clothes and hope no one will notice! Some rely on The Genesis 3:12 Defense and blame others for their behavior. Some don't eat anything for two days before their First Place 4 Health weigh-in and then go out for a celebration meal once the meeting is over. Some even choose not to go to their First Place 4 Health meeting rather than face the truth!

As you write your folly story, try to make it humorous but also make it factual—the point is to be honest. God already knows your folly—and you do, too—so there is no sense in trying to hide from the truth! Write in your spiritual journal for privacy!

O Lord God, how silly I must look to You when I go to great lengths to cover my sin rather than go to great lengths to obey Your Word! Forgive me for my folly, and according to Your promise, forgive my sins when I come to You in contrite confession. Amen.

REFLECTION AND APPLICATION

Day 7

Loving Lord, thank You for forgiving my sins and making me a new creation in Christ Jesus. As a new creation, I need to learn new ways and think new thoughts. Help me to learn those newness lessons today. Amen.

During yesterday's time of reflection and application, you wrote a folly story, a personal account of a time you tried to hide your sin from God and others. Today, having confessed that folly to God, you are ready to leave that painful incident behind. It's time to go back to the scene of the crime and replay the tape, this time with a much different ending.

Recall the situation that led you into temptation; then in your journal, rewrite the story to illustrate how the new, forgiven you would do things differently—a "right-way instant replay." Perhaps you will need to picture yourself avoiding the pastry aisle and concentrating your shopping efforts on the perimeter of the store. Maybe you will pass up the magazine that contains the latest fad diet because you are committed to the First Place 4 Health program. Instead of buying the magazine, picture treating yourself to a piece of fresh fruit that is usually outside your food budget. Instead of visualizing the larger-sized clothing you purchased to hide your indulgence, see yourself shopping in the regular-sized clothing department! Feel the joy of seeing the number go down at your next weigh-in.

Once you have envisioned what success feels like, take that attitude into the new day the Lord has created for your enjoyment. In Jesus Christ, you are forgiven. There is no need to carry your past sins or allow their memory to weigh you down.

There is no sin too great for You to forgive, O Lord, no folly outside the bounds of Your mercy, compassion and love. Thank You for loving me enough to send Jesus to die for me so that I can live for You. Amen.

Group Prayer Requests

first place 4 health

Today's Date: ____________________

Name	Request

Results

____

____

____

____

____

____

____

Week Six

God's truth and temptation's lie

Scripture Memory Verse

No temptation has seized you except what is common to man. And God is faithful; he will not let you be tempted beyond what you can bear. But when you are tempted, he will also provide a way out so that you can stand up under it.

1 Corinthians 10:13

"Pray that you will not fall into temptation" was one of the last commands that the Lord Jesus gave His disciples before He was crucified (Luke 22:40; see also Matthew 26:41; Mark 14:38). Yet, in typical human fashion, Jesus' disciples were much too busy trying to figure out who would be the greatest in God's kingdom to heed their Master's advice.

All too soon the folly of not doing what Jesus had commanded became clear: When temptation came, all the disciples deserted Jesus, leaving Him to face the final agonizing moments of His life here on Earth without the love and support of those He had loved and supported for three long years. The disciples had just been with Jesus in the Upper Room. They had shared a meal with Him and heard His final words of instruction. When Jesus tried to warn them about what was about to take place, they all vowed that they were ready to go to death and prison with Jesus. But when put to the test, their boasting words turned into blatant denial of the One they vowed to serve.

Something we learned about on Day Six of our Week Four study happened. The disciples had made a commitment to Jesus, and what was lurking right outside the door? Temptation had predictably followed their promises of faithfulness.

When you enrolled in this session of First Place 4 Health and began this *Begin with Christ* Bible study, what commitment did you make? How have you seen the "temptation always follows commitment" pattern play itself out in your life since beginning this session of First Place 4 Health? How has temptation reared its ugly head?

If the temptation that predictably follows commitment were the end of the story, we would have no reason for hope. But praise be to God, He never leaves us to face our problems alone!

Day 1

JESUS WAS TEMPTED

O Lord God Almighty, I know that Jesus was tempted just like I am, yet He always did what is pleasing to You. Give me wisdom and insight as I look to Jesus and learn from Him. Amen.

In our Day Three study during Week Two, we learned about Jesus, our great high priest. In that lesson, we learned that Jesus was "tempted in every way, just as we are–yet was without sin" (Hebrews 4:15). Now it's easy to look at verses like that and say, "Yes, but Jesus was God! Of course, He didn't sin. But I'm human; I can't be expected to resist temptation."

When we say that, though, we have fallen for Satan's lie! In a mystery too great for our finite minds to possibly comprehend, Jesus was fully divine–God in human flesh–and He was also fully human. His temptations were every bit as real as ours. If that were not true, our great high priest would not be able to sympathize with us in our weaknesses. Jesus was tempted. He felt the same emotions we feel when being enticed by the evil one. As a result, we can follow Jesus' example when we are looking for a way to escape temptation, because He has shown us the way.

Immediately after Jesus was baptized by John in the Jordan River, heaven opened and two amazing things happened. Turn to Matthew 3:16-17 in your Bible, and record what two things happened that day.

The Holy Spirit anointed Jesus for the ministry He had been chosen to fulfill, and God the Father affirmed that Jesus was His Son, the Son whom He loved and with whom He was well pleased. What an exciting moment that must have been! But no sooner had that happened when another event occurred: Jesus was tempted. Matthew begins the narrative of Jesus' temptation with a sentence that at first seems contradictory. Turn to Matthew 4:1. Matthew tells us:

Then __________ was __________ by the __________ into the __________ to be __________ by the __________.

We are told that the Spirit led Jesus into the desert. Was this wilderness trip something that was against God's will? Why or why not?

Even though the Spirit led Jesus into the desert to be tested, who actually did the tempting?

As we will discover during our next few days of study, Jesus successfully withstood the devil's wiles. We could say that He passed the test with flying colors; He aced the test. What does the fact that the Spirit led Jesus into the desert to be tempted tell you about the purpose of temptation from God's perspective? Is it an opportunity to succeed or an invitation to fail? Think this question through before you answer.

God tests us to build up our faith, to show that we are sincere in our commitment, to confirm that our eyes are fixed on Jesus. Satan, on the other hand, uses temptation to lure us into failure. Think now about the last time you were tempted. Did you prove yourself faithful to your First Place 4 Health commitment, or did you succumb to Satan's wiles, and if so, why?

If you did not stand firm in your faith, confess this failing to God and receive His forgiveness so that you do not have to carry the burden of this failure with you into tomorrow's study.

O gracious Lord, thank You for forgiving me when I fail. Because of Your tender mercy, I can begin each new day without having to drag my past behind me. Amen.

Day 2 A PREDICTABLE PATTERN

O Lord, my comfort in my suffering is this: Your promise preserves my life. Amen (Psalm 119:50).

Not only is commitment followed by temptation a predictable pattern, but also Satan uses a predictable pattern when attempting to lead us astray. Today we will look at the way the devil tempted Jesus and how Jesus responded so that we too can be prepared to withstand Satan's trickery.

Matthew 4:2 gives us a valuable clue to one of Satan's predictable patterns. What do we learn about Jesus in this verse?

____

____

____

Jesus was hungry—not just a little hungry, but famished! He had been fasting for 40 days and 40 nights. What did the tempter come to Jesus and say? Verse 3 of Matthew 4 has the answer.

______ you are the ________ of ________, tell these ________ to become ________.

Satan used Jesus' physical weakness to tempt Him to turn the stones into bread, to use His God-given power to satisfy His own physical hunger. But before Satan mentioned food, what did the tempter question?

____

____

How is the phrase "If you are the Son of God" like the serpent's question to Eve that fateful day in the garden? (Refer to Day One of our Week Five study to help you remember what the serpent said to Eve and what the tempter's words implied.)

Satan always begins his temptation by inviting us to question God's goodness and love. The evil one would like for us to believe that God is withholding something from us that we need in order to be whole and complete. "Did God really say . . ." "If you are a beloved child of God, why is your heavenly Father treating you this way?" Can you hear the sarcasm in the evil one's voice, even as you read these words? Stop for a moment and consider how feelings of deprivation are often the means Satan uses to tempt you to eat something outside the boundaries of your Live It plan. What did you discover?

Whenever you hear a voice that questions God's goodness, love, ongoing provision or continuing protection, what should you immediately do? (The answer was in the introduction to this week's study.)

Jesus shows us something else we can do when our archenemy comes calling. According to Matthew 4:4, how did Jesus answer Satan's taunt?

Jesus countered Satan's lie with a direct quote from the Word of God—word for word, as found in Deuteronomy 8:3! How is the way Jesus answered Satan's lie different from the way Eve replied?

What new behavior do you learn from today's study? What behavior will better equip you to stand firm the next time you are tempted?

Our memory verse tells us that God will provide a way out when we are tempted. How did God provide a way out of temptation for His beloved Son?

God's Word and prayer are your first lines of defense, too! Use them often and well.

O God, thank You for giving me Your Word as an assurance of Your love and provision. Thank You that I can defend myself against Satan's wiles when I counter his attack with Scripture I have memorized for such a time. Amen.

Day 3

A REPEAT PERFORMANCE

Thank You, Lord, for Your precious Word. Help me to rely on Your provision and not on my own wit when I find myself being tempted by the enemy. Amen.

Yesterday we watched Jesus defend Himself against the temptation to satisfy His legitimate hunger in an illegitimate way. Jesus had been sent to Earth to minister to God's people, not to use His power to satisfy His own wants. Jesus lived a life of total dependence on His Father in heaven for the provision of His every need.

How might Satan tempt you to fill a legitimate need in an illegitimate way when you are hungry?

Jesus did not give in to Satan's lure. Instead, He stood firm in His commitment to carry out the plan and purpose for which He had been anointed by the Spirit. When you indulge your appetite rather than follow Jesus' example and stand firmly on the Word of God, how might you be missing out on the plan and purpose God has for you? (You might want to write your thoughts in your journal.)

When Satan's first attempt failed, Matthew tells us that Satan staged an almost instant replay, a repeat performance with slight variations. Satan is always persistent in his efforts to lead God's people astray. What does that tell you about our need to be persistent, too?

Our memory verse for this week tells us about something we have that Satan lacks: God's protection and God's great and precious promises. What has God promised to provide for you?

The first time Satan tempted Jesus, the tempter enticed Jesus to satisfy His legitimate physical hunger in an inappropriate way. The second time, Satan upped the ante. In fact, not only did Satan up the ante, he did so by misrepresenting the Word of God! Turn to Matthew 4:5-7 in your Bible, and read the account of Jesus' second temptation. When Satan spoke to Jesus the second time, what did the tempter first say (verse 6)?

Those same words were at the beginning of the first temptation, too. Satan was once again trying to plant doubt in Jesus' mind. However, this time the temptation was not to satisfy Jesus' need for physical food. This time Jesus was asked to prove that God would protect His Son, even if Jesus did something contrary to His Father's revealed Word: first provision, next protection. Satan knows our human insecurities well!

Satan even quoted a portion of God's Word, Psalm 91:11-12, as part of his deception. However, the archenemy pulled those two verses out of context; he separated them from the whole counsel of God. Jesus' answer shows us the error of Satan's reasoning. What did Jesus say as He quoted Deuteronomy 6:16?

It is also written: "________ not put the ____________ your __________ to the test."

How do you test God when you do things that have the potential to damage your body—things like overeating and under-exercising—and then expect God to protect you and keep you from illness and harm?

Why do you think reading large portions of Scripture, studying the Bible and memorizing key verses are an important trio of defense?

Thank You, Loving Lord, for showing me the way to resist the devil. I will read Your Word daily so that I will not be thrown off base by Satan's deception. Amen.

THREE'S A CHARM

Day 4

Lord God, You know me better than I know myself. You know that I am easily deceived by Satan's lies. Thank You for eyes to see the truth, and the courage to stand firm in the face of temptation. Amen.

For the past two days, we have learned how the devil tried to persuade Jesus to abandon Christ's God-given purpose in favor of instant gratification. What new information that will help you counter Satan's attacks have you learned from this week's studies?

When Jesus didn't succumb to the devil's first two temptations, Satan reappeared, this time with a third offer. Jesus had not provided food for Himself, even though He was hungry. Jesus did not put His Father to the test in an attempt to prove God really did love and value Him. Surely, Satan reasoned, Jesus would opt for instant power! Go back to Matthew 4, and read verses 8-10. What did Satan offer Jesus, and what would Jesus need to do to obtain it?

Were all the kingdoms of the world Satan's to give? (You might want to look at Psalm 24:1-2 before answering this question.)

Satan was offering Jesus something that was not his to give away! And in that fact, we find another characteristic of temptation we can be on the lookout for. Temptation always offers us something appealing that it cannot give us; it offers to satisfy a need, but it does not have the means or substance to deliver.

How do diet and exercise programs that offer instant results promise us something appealing, when, in fact, they cannot deliver what they have advertised?

You might want to reflect on a time you fell for an instant-result, quick-fix weight-loss solution before you answer this question.

Jesus answered Satan with another Scripture verse, this one from Deuteronomy 6:13: "Worship the Lord your God, and serve him only." But this time around Jesus did more than just quote Scripture. What else did our Lord say to Satan (see Matthew 4:10)?

Jesus told Satan, "Away from me." Later, Jesus' brother James would write, "Submit yourselves, then, to God. Resist the devil and he will flee from you" (James 4:7). What can you learn from these words that will help you in your First Place 4 Health efforts?

Sadly, all too often we submit to Satan's temptation and resist God's Word! What have you learned in today's lesson that will help you break that downward cycle? Give a very practical example of a new temptation-busting tool you have acquired this week.

Thank God for providing a way of escape when temptation comes, because the Father has sent Jesus to Earth to show you the way!

Great God, You do provide a way out for me when I am tempted. Help me to have eyes to see the escape You have provided so that I can draw near to You and find strength in my time of need. Amen.

MINISTERING ANGELS

Day 5

Thank You, gracious Lord, that when I have endured temptation for a while, You will provide me with comfort and rest. Amen.

After three attempts to thwart Jesus' mission, Satan left Jesus alone. Although Matthew does not record this particular detail, Luke tells us, "When the devil had finished all this tempting, he left him until an opportune time" (Luke 4:13). What do those words tell you about the nature of Satan and temptation?

Satan is an opportunist, an enemy who always strikes when we are vulnerable. Sometimes that vulnerability is caused by physical weakness, but often we are most vulnerable when we have just withstood one test and are feeling proud. When we least expect it, Satan slips in and catches us with our guard down. How does our memory verse describe what temptation does?

What images does the word "seized" bring up for you?

Even though Satan is crafty, persistent and deceptive, our God is faithful. How does our memory verse describe God's faithfulness?

How have you experienced God's faithfulness when you have been about to succumb to temptation this week? Make your answer relevant to First Place 4 Health.

Matthew 4:11 tells us that when the devil left Jesus, someone came and attended Him. Who did God send to comfort Jesus?

How might the other members of your First Place 4 Health group be part of God's faithful provision to help you find a way out of temptation and to comfort you when you have gone through a season of testing? Be specific in the ways your First Place 4 Health group has attended to you when you were in need of strength and encouragement.

Often we do not realize when God has used us as His special messengers, sent to bring comfort to those who are suffering. Write a note thanking one of your special, God-sent "angels," telling that person what his or her care and concern have meant to you.

Having written to one of your human encouragers, now take up your spiritual journal and spend time thanking God for providing you with a way out when you are being tempted by the evil one.

Thank You for Your faithfulness and love, O Lord. Thank You for friends who are making this journey with me, friends who can give me strength and encouragement so that I can resist the wiles of the devil. Amen.

REFLECTION AND APPLICATION

Day 6

O Lord God, I have hidden Your Word in my heart so that I will not sin against You. Amen.
(Psalm 119:11)

This week we have been learning about God's faithfulness and Satan's lies. As we have seen, in order to successfully resist the devil, we must first understand the nature of temptation.

The first thing we need to realize about temptation is that it is always a solicitation to fill a legitimate need in an illegitimate way. We also need to know that temptation always promises something it can't deliver. Temptation is like putting a fake worm on a hook and dangling it in front of a fish. The fish is hungry, and hunger is a legitimate need. However, that a plastic worm can satisfy that need is only a pretense. The invitation is, "Come and bite into this juicy worm. Have an easy snack. Why don't you just try it? You'll never really know how delicious it is until you take the first bite." And before the fish knows it—*Wham!*—the fish is in the net. That's what temptation does to us, too. Temptation is always an invitation to fill a legitimate need in an illegitimate way.

For those of us committed to the First Place 4 Health program, the ongoing temptation to satisfy our legitimate hunger by eating something that does not support our commitment to health and balance is a constant danger. Temptation entices us to grab a sugary snack for quick energy rather than prepare a nutritious meal that will truly sustain our tired bodies. And for a quick minute, we do feel energized as the sugar surges through our bloodstream.

Soon, however, the devil is laughing and sneering at us, mocking us for our foolishness. Not only have we crashed physically as the sugar high wears off, but we are also berating ourselves for being so gullible. After all, we knew better when we took that first bite! We knew that candy bar was promising something it could not deliver. Satan is the father of lies. He is behind the temptations that promise to satisfy legitimate needs in illegitimate ways. God has promised to supply all our needs with good things that bring lasting satisfaction. And our faithful God has also promised to give us a way out of temptation. Our challenge is to resist the devil and stand firm in our faith.

What have you learned about temptation this week that will help you stand firm in your commitment to health, wholeness, balance and a lifestyle that pleases God? Each day's lesson contained one or more truths to equip you before you are seized by temptation.

In the space below, list as many truths to stand firm on as you can. (Perhaps reviewing your daily work will help you recall all we studied this week.)

Gracious God, thank You for Your faithfulness and love. You have given me all I need to live a life pleasing to You, and I am grateful for Your provision. Amen.

Day 7 REFLECTION AND APPLICATION

O LORD, the God who saves me, day and night I cry out before You. May my prayer come before You; turn Your ear to my cry. Amen (Psalm 88:1).

During yesterday's reflection and application time, you were asked to make a list of the things you have learned during this week's study about the ways you can stand firm against temptation. Today we are going to make another list, this one about God's faithfulness. Drawing from all that you have studied thus far in the *Begin with Christ* Bible study, list what you have learned about God's faithfulness. The items on your list can include new information you have gleaned from this study and prior knowledge that has been reconfirmed so that you realize the truth in a deeper level of your being. You can use the lines below or write your list in your spiritual journal.

After making your list of the ways God has revealed His faithfulness to you, spend the rest of your time praising God for all His wonderful mercies. He is indeed faithful!

Great is Your faithfulness! Your mercies are new every morning and your compassion is without end. How grateful I am that You are my God and I am Your precious, beloved child. Amen.

Group Prayer Requests

Today's Date: ______________________

Name	Request

Results

Week Seven

spiritual food for spiritual life

Scripture Memory Verse

Man does not live on bread alone,

but on every word that comes from the mouth of God.

Matthew 4:4

Last week we learned how Jesus Christ, the example we can always look to, faced temptation in the desert wilderness. On three different occasions, Satan came to our Savior with a very tempting offer. And three times Jesus said, "It is written . . ." What was Jesus referring to when He used those words? What was written?

Now stop and think about where God's Word was written during Jesus' wilderness testing. Jesus did not have a bunch of parchment scrolls out in the desert with Him when Satan appeared to test Him. And this was obviously long before the days of handheld wireless computers or instant messages. Where was God's Word written?

What does that tell you about the importance of memorizing the Scripture verses that correspond with each of your First Place 4 Health weekly Bible studies?

Members who have been in First Place 4 Health for many years have an inner storehouse that is chock-full of God's Word. These First Place 4 Health veterans report time after time when the Holy Spirit was able to draw out just the verse they needed when they needed it, because they had been faithful to memorize God's Word and hide it in their hearts. That same benefit can be yours, so be diligent to do your Scripture memory work!

THE BREAD OF LIFE

Day 1

O loving and gracious Lord, You are the bread of life, the One who came to Earth to die for my sins so that I would have eternal life in You. Amen.

During Day Four of our Week Two study, you were given a list of "I Am" statements to complete. One of those "I Am" verses was John 6:48. Turn to that verse in your Bible and complete the verse again.

I ________ the ________________ of ____________.

Jesus also said those same words in John 6:35, except in this verse He gave us more information. What else did Jesus tell us?

I am the bread of life. ________ who ____________ to __________ will never go ______________,
and ________ who ______________ in me will ______________ be ______________.

Because we do not understand the original language of the writer, these statements might seem confusing. Certainly those who believe in Jesus still need physical food to eat and physical water to drink. In the physical realm, food, water, air and shelter are basic necessities that sustain life. But Jesus is not talking about food and water in the physical realm. In Greek (the language the New Testament was written in), there are three different words that are translated into our English word "life." It is important that we understand the difference between the three.

bios = biological, or physical, life

Turn to Mark 4:19 to read an example of "life" translated from *bios*. What is Mark telling us about life in this verse?

____

____

____

psuche = self-life, or mental/emotional life

Our self-life—our ego—is mentioned in Luke 14:26. What does this verse tell us we must be prepared to do with our self-life (ego) if we are to become disciples of Jesus?

zoe = God's life, or spiritual life

According to John 10:10, Jesus said, "I have come that they may have life, and have it to the full." Which type of life do you think Jesus was referring to here and in John 6:35, the verse you wrote out near the beginning of today's lesson?

Now go back and add the word "spiritual" before the word "life." This will help you understand the truth Jesus is imparting to His disciples.

First Place 4 Health addresses all three meanings of the word "life." First, how does First Place 4 Health deal with our *bios*, or physical life?

How does First Place 4 Health deal with our *psuche*, or ego-driven self-life?

How does First Place 4 Health address our *zoe*, or spiritual life?

What happens when these three forms of life are at war within us—when our *bios*, our *psuche* and our *zoe* are not in agreement with one another?

What would happen if we were doing something harmful to our biological self? How would our spiritual self, the part that longs to please God, react?

How might the fact that your spiritual life was not being nourished explain why the diet and exercise programs you participated in before coming to First Place 4 Health were destined to fail?

We can't dissect ourselves into three parts, each operating independently of the other two, so how does knowing about the different types of life mentioned in the Bible help you understand the importance of the balance and wholeness of the First Place 4 Health program?

O Father, You have created me in complex ways that are beyond my comprehension. Yet Your instructions to me are really simple. You ask that I love You with all my heart, all my mind, all my heart and all my spirit. Amen.

Day 2 YOU MUST BE BORN AGAIN!

O gracious and compassionate Lord, today I pray for eyes to see, ears to hear and a heart that is eager to understand the truth of Your Word. Amen.

Yesterday we learned why it is important to differentiate between the different types of life when we strive to properly interpret Jesus' words. There was another fellow in Scripture who was confused because he failed to differentiate between the truths of the physical realm, the mental/emotional realm and the spiritual realm. Turn to John 3:1-18 in your Bible. What was this man's name and what was his confusion?

____

____

____

Obviously, on the physical plane, this man was correct. We cannot be born again. But on the spiritual plane, we *must* be born again. According to John 3:3, what can't we do until we have been born again spiritually?

____

____

____

Our memory verse for Week Two dealt with the kingdom of God. How is being spiritually born again part of the First Place 4 Health program?

____

____

____

John 3:5 tells us what the second birth is about. Jesus prefaced His explanation:

__________ tell __________ the __________.

What does the presence of these words tell you about the importance of this teaching?

____

____

____

What did Jesus tell us we must be born of this second time?

And in order to be "born of water and the Spirit," we must each do something that is very important. John 3:16-18 tells us what that essential step is. Read these verses, and then summarize Jesus' teaching in your own words.

According to John 3:12, Jesus told Nicodemus that there was a connection between Jesus' earthly teaching and heavenly things. Paraphrase what Jesus said.

In First Place 4 Health, we learn about physical things—and we learn about spiritual things, too. Think about applying John 3:12 to our First Place 4 Health program. Can we learn about spiritual things if we are not willing to be obedient to Jesus in the physical realm? Why or why not? Think your answer through before you write it down!

How does this truth combat Satan's lie that tells us we can grow spiritually while our physical self is out of control?

One of the central themes of First Place 4 Health is *balance*. How do Jesus' words in John 3:12 address balance, grasping truth in both the physical and the spiritual realms?

If you excel in one or two areas of your First Place 4 Health program but are negligent of the other areas, what is your life lacking?

How might Jesus' words in John 3:12 be applicable to that problem?

Do you think the eternal life Jesus spoke of in John 3:16 is physical life (*bios*), self-life (*psuche*) or spiritual life (*zoe*), and why?

Lord Jesus, You are the light of the world. Thank You for bringing me out of darkness and into Your marvelous light. You surely deserve first place in the new life You have given me. Amen.

Day 3

JESUS IS THE GATEWAY

Lord Jesus, You took on all my sins, everything I have ever done wrong, so that I could be right with God. I will express my gratitude by caring for myself because You care so much for me! Amen.

Another of the "I Am" statements you completed in Day Four of the Week Two study is found in John 10:9. Turn to John 10 in your Bible, and read verses 7-10.

According to verses 7 and 9, Jesus referred to Himself as "the gate." Obviously, Jesus was not talking about a physical gate, something made of wood or metal designed to give access or exit to and from an enclosed area. Once again, we will not understand Jesus' teaching if we try to understand that what is being said refers to the physical plane.

According to verse 9, after declaring Himself the gate, Jesus said something else. What happens to the one who enters through Him?

Belief in Jesus is the gateway that gives entrance into God's kingdom; it is the gate that gives us safe passage into eternal life. How is the life Jesus came to give us described in John 10:10?

Was Jesus talking about physical life or spiritual life, and why do you believe that is true?

All the riches of God the Father and all the power of God the Holy Spirit only become available to us through Jesus, the gateway that gives us entrance into God's kingdom. Think back to the Week Two memory verse, which is the main verse for the First Place 4 Health program. What is it that we are to seek, and how is Jesus, the gateway, part of that seeking?

Jesus also said that "the thief" tries to block our entrance into the Good Shepherd's fold. What does the thief come to do (see John 10:10)?

How is this different from the benefits we receive when we enter God's eternal kingdom through Jesus Christ, the only way to the Father? Explain your answer thoroughly.

According to John 10:11, what did Jesus tell us He is, and what did He come to do?

Reflect for a moment on Day Three of the Week Five study, in which we learned that God had to do something to cover Adam's and Eve's nakedness. What did God have to do to cover their sin?

As we learned in our Week Five studies, that same sin covering is available to us today. But God no longer has to sacrifice an animal to cover our transgressions. Explain why this is so.

Thank You, Lord God, for sending Jesus to take on my sins. In and through Him, You are no longer counting my sins against me. I am forgiven. Praise God! Amen.

Day 4

BELIEVE IN HIM!

O Lord, You promise me that when I confess with my mouth that Jesus is Lord and believe in my heart that God raised Him from the dead, I will be saved. Amen (Romans 10:9).

Thus far this week, we have looked at Jesus, the bread of life, the gateway that gives us access to the Father's love and the Spirit's power. God has done everything that He must do to make the kingdom of God a reality for us. When Jesus stretched out His arms on the cross and declared, "It is finished," there was nothing else that needed to be done (John 19:30). Jesus had accomplished His mission; He had saved His people from their sins by dying in their place. Three days later, Jesus rose from the tomb and ascended into heaven to sit at God the Father's right hand.

What is the resurrected Lord Jesus doing for us even as we complete this First Place 4 Health study? (See Hebrews 7:24-25 if you need help with the answer.)

____

____

____

Hebrews 7:25 tells us about something special that Jesus can do:

> He is able to save ____________ those who come to __________ through ____________, because he ____________ ____________ to ____________ for them.

How does this truth correspond to what we learned yesterday about Jesus being the gateway?

____

____

____

When Jesus died on the cross of Calvary, God's plan for our eternal salvation was complete. Jesus put to death all our sins so that we could be made right with God. But there is one thing we must do to inherit eternal life. Turn to Acts 16 and read what Paul and Silas told the man who asked, "Sirs, what must I do to be saved?" (verse 30). According to verse 31, what did Paul and Silas tell the man?

____

____

____

____

With that answer comes another question, this time a very personal question: Do you believe that the Lord Jesus Christ is the only way to a right relationship with God the Father? Do you believe that Jesus, the Messiah, took on all your sins in order to reconcile you to God? Thoroughly explain your answer.

If in answering the last question you discovered that you do not believe in your heart that Jesus is both your Lord and Savior, take a moment to make that profession right now. Revelation 3:20 tells us that Jesus is standing at the door of your heart. He is knocking, asking that you allow Him to be the Lord of your life. Are you ready to make that bold confession right now?

Perhaps you made a public profession that Jesus was your Lord and Savior many years ago, but through this *Begin with Christ* Bible study, you have come to accept Jesus as the way, the truth and the life at a deeper level. The profession you made years ago has become a living reality, not just words you said way back then. If that is your situation, you, too, can benefit from renewing your commitment to Jesus Christ as your Savior.

If you are ready to take this all-important step right now, pray the following prayer in the stillness of your heart:

> *Gracious and loving Father, I humbly confess that I have broken Your laws, and my sins have separated me from You. I am truly sorry, and I want to turn away from my past sinful life so that I can turn toward You. Please forgive me, and help me avoid sinning again. I believe that Your Son, Jesus Christ, died for my sins, was resurrected from the dead, is alive and hears my prayers. I invite Jesus to become the Lord of my life, to rule and reign in my heart from this day forward. Please send Your Holy Spirit to help me hear Your voice and obey Your commands. It is my desire to do Your will and bring honor and glory to You in all I say and do. In Jesus' name I pray. Amen.*

Once you have accepted Jesus as your Lord and Savior, it is important that you share the good news with your First Place 4 Health group leader, a pastor or another mature Christian. He or she will be able to pray with and for you and guide you as you make a connection with a local church where you can be nurtured in your new faith. If you have not been baptized, make arrangements to do that soon. Baptism is an outward sign of the inner new birth you have just experienced. Luke 15:10 tells us there is rejoicing in heaven when one sinner repents. The angels are rejoicing with you right now. Welcome to the great and wonderful kingdom of God!

How will your new life in Christ help you as you complete this First Place 4 Health Bible study?

Father, thank You for hearing my prayer and accepting my confession that Jesus Christ is my Savior and my Lord. Thank You for the new life that begins the moment I confess Jesus Christ as the One who saves me from my life of sin. Amen.

THE LIVING WORD

Day 5

O Jesus, You are the bread of life.
When I feast on You, my soul will be satisfied. Amen.

In the prologue to the Gospel of John, the apostle gives us some more important information about this man Jesus Christ, the Savior and Lord we strive to keep first in all things. Turn to John 1:1-5 and prayerfully read these wonderful words. What is John saying in these verses? Write in your own words what John says.

Verse 4 tells us:

In ______ was ______, and that ______ was the ______ of men.

Which one of the "I Am" statements recorded on Day Four of our Week Two study does John 1:5 correspond to? Reread John 8:12, and compare it to John 1:5.

John 1:2 tells us where the Word was in the beginning. Where was the Word?

Genesis 1:1-26 describes the creation of the world. How was the Word part of the miracle of creation?

How does John 1:3 describe the same thing that Genesis 1:1-26 describes?

Now look at John 1:14. What did this same Word that was present and active in the creation of the world do?

The Word became ______________ and ____________ ________
______________ among ________.

John 1:14 describes the One who became flesh and dwelt among us for a while, called by a name other than "Word." Who does John 1:14 tell us this living Word is?

If Jesus is the living Word of God, the same Word that brought forth creation, how powerful are the words He speaks?

How does the fact that Jesus is the living Word also better explain our memory verse for this week?

John 1:14 tells us two things about Jesus:

Jesus was "full of ______ and ______."

How does this fact affirm the truth that He can "completely" save us (see Hebrews 7:25)?

Because Jesus, the living Word, is also the bread of life, what happens when we eat this spiritual bread?

How does this help you better understand why daily Bible study, Scripture reading and Scripture memory work are such an important part of the First Place 4 Health program?

What is the connection between what we eat in the physical realm and the amount of spiritual food we eat? Explain your answer thoroughly.

Thank You, loving Father, for sending Jesus, the living Word, so that my soul will never be hungry or thirsty again. Amen.

Day 6

REFLECTION AND APPLICATION

O Lord God, I will seek You while You can be found, knowing that to put off until tomorrow what You ask me to do today is not part of my First Place 4 Health program. Amen.

On Sunday night, October 8, 1871, the famous evangelist Dwight L. Moody gave a fiery sermon to a standing-room-only crowd. The service was held at Farwell Hall, rather than Moody's church, to accommodate the large crowd in attendance that night. At the conclusion of the message, Moody gave the people a charge to go home and think about what had been said, and the need to accept Jesus Christ as their personal Lord and Savior. Dwight ended his message by saying he would ask the people to come forward, make a commitment and receive Christ when they returned the following week. But, sadly, that crowd never had an opportunity to meet the following week. Even as the closing song was being sung that fateful night, the din of fire trucks and church bells announced that Chicago was on fire. Many of those present that night perished in the flames. After that experience, Dwight Moody vowed never again to postpone asking people to commit their lives to Christ and confess Him as their Lord and Savior.

Centuries before Dwight Moody's vow, the prophet Isaiah told God's people to "seek the LORD while he may be found; call on him while he is near"—to reach out to God while there is the opportunity to do so (Isaiah 55:6). Tomorrow is not guaranteed.

This week, our *Begin with Christ* lessons have invited those of us who have not previously made a commitment to Jesus Christ to do so. Those who had already professed Jesus as their Lord and Savior were invited to renew that vow, especially if they have experienced Jesus in new, vibrant ways through this Bible study. If you were reluctant to plunge into the Living Water earlier in the week, it is not too late to do so. Simply turn back to the Day Four study and confess your belief in Jesus, the One who came to save you from your sins.

Almighty and sovereign Lord, thank You for giving me the courage to make a commitment to Jesus Christ as my Lord and Savior. He died for me. Help me to live for Him. Amen.

REFLECTION AND APPLICATION

Day 7

O Lord, I know that I do not live by physical bread alone. My spiritual nourishment comes from the living Word that sustains my soul. Amen.

We have now passed the halfway point in our *Begin with Christ* Bible study, and we have covered a lot of territory! Today will truly be a day of reflection as we remember what we have learned thus far. To the right of each of the Week headings in the chart on the following page, list something you learned from that week's study that you were able to successfully apply to your First Place 4 Health efforts. After listing what you learned, tell how you have been able to apply that learning in a way that contributed to the health and balance of the First Place 4 Health program.

Be prepared to share this information with your First Place 4 Health group this week so that they, too, can benefit from what God has taught you during this *Begin with Christ* Bible study.

Thank You, Lord, for lessons learned and for a wonderful First Place 4 Health group that I can share my insights with, even as I also learn from them. Amen.

WEEK	Something new I learned that has made a positive difference in my First Place 4 Health efforts:	How I have applied that learning to my First Place 4 Health program:
Two		
Three		
Four		
Five		
Six		
Seven		

Group Prayer Requests

first place 4 health

Today's Date: ______________________

Name	Request

Results

Week Eight

radical transformation

Scripture Memory Verse

Do not conform any longer to the pattern of this world, but be transformed by the renewing of your mind. Then you will be able to test and approve what God's will is—his good, pleasing and perfect will.

Romans 12:2

We live in an instant-gratification society: instant food, instant messages, instant intimacy and instant success. And because we have been conditioned by the immediate-gratification mentality of the world we live in, we have continually gravitated to diet and exercise programs that promise instant results. Never mind the fact we needed to lose 100 pounds; we were told we could start the diet in September and have the body we'd always dreamed of by the holidays! Visions of a sleek body danced through our head as we signed on the dotted line–and we imagined ourselves transformed in the twinkling of an eye.

Sadly, in our desire for the instantaneous, we let go of the possible. We were looking for instant perfection rather than a gradual process of transformation. In our haste to achieve our quick-fix goals, we forgot that God is not interested in instant results. God is in the business of building character, and building character takes time.

"Exactly how much time does the journey to health and wholeness take?" we impatiently ask. When we look to Scripture for an answer to the "how long" question, God's answer is very clear: The process of transformation begins the moment we accept Jesus Christ as our Lord and Savior and continues until that glorious day when we are taken up to heaven to be with our Lord forever. This spiritual journey we are on is about putting off the old and putting on the new–replacing our old destructive habits with a new lifestyle that promotes balance and wholeness. In theological terms, that lifelong process is called sanctification. God simply calls it transformation as He does His good work in us moment by moment, day by day, over the course of a lifetime.

RENEW YOUR MIND

Day 1

Gracious and loving Lord, You ask that I offer myself as a living sacrifice to You. Thank You that I can trust in You rather than rely on the world's wisdom as I undertake to live and move and have my being in You. Amen.

Because we are four-sided beings, our renewal efforts must take place in all four aspects of our person. We must renew our spirits, our bodies, our emotions and our minds. And although all four aspects are somewhat separate, they are also interconnected. Our brain, the marvelous organ where our thought life is processed, is really part of our physical body. Our emotions are a combination of our thoughts and the chemical reactions they produce in our body. Our spirit is often burdened by what is going on in our physical body, our thought life and our emotions.

What does this tell you about the importance of renewing all four aspects of your being in a balanced manner?

Our memory verse for this week speaks about the renewal of one specific aspect of our being. What does our memory verse talk about renewing?

What do the words "do not conform any longer" imply?

What was it we used to conform to?

Once our mind has been renewed, what will we be able to do?

According to our memory verse, is it possible to discern God's will—"his good, pleasing and perfect will"—when we are still conforming to the way of the world? Explain your answer.

Can those who are still stuck in the instant-gratification mentality of the world we live in discern God's will? Why or why not?

Proverbs 3:5 tells us: "Trust in the LORD with all your heart and lean not on your own understanding." How is leaning on our understanding like conforming to the pattern of this world?

When we trust in the Lord with all our heart, what will we be able to test and approve, and why is that important to our success in First Place 4 Health?

Lord God Almighty, forgive me for those times I expect instant results when Your good, pleasing and perfect will is that I be transformed through this lifelong process called renewal. Amen.

TRANSFORMED FROM THE INSIDE OUT

Day 2

O Lord, thank You that when I fix my eyes on You,
I am transformed by the power of Your Holy Spirit in
accordance with Your great eternal plan and purpose. Amen.

Whenever we are trying to comprehend a particular passage in God's Word, it is often helpful to read several translations and paraphrases of that text to enrich our understanding. This is especially true of our memory verse for this week.

Begin today's study by writing this week's memory verse as it appears in the *New International Version,* which is the translation used in our First Place 4 Health Bible studies.

Eugene Peterson, in his Scripture paraphrase titled *THE MESSAGE,* words Romans 12:2 like this:

> *Don't become so well-adjusted to your culture that you fit into it without even thinking. Instead, fix your attention on God. You'll be changed from the inside out. Readily recognize what he wants from you, and quickly respond to it. Unlike the culture around you, always dragging you down to its level of immaturity, God brings the best out of you, develops well-formed maturity in you.*

In what ways have you become so "well-adjusted" to our instant-results society that you have expected to repair the damage caused by many years of out-of-control eating in one quick-fix season of intense diet and exercise?

According to *THE MESSAGE*, how are we changed when we fix our attention on God?

According to *THE MESSAGE,* you are to "recognize what [God] wants from you, and quickly respond to it." What have you recognized that God wants from you through this *Begin with Christ* Bible study?

Have you responded to God's request quickly, or are you still putting off until tomorrow what God asks you to do today? Explain your answer.

According to *THE MESSAGE* version of Romans 12:2, what does the culture around us do to us?

In contrast to the culture around us, what does God do for us?

How is your participation in the First Place 4 Health program bringing the best out of you?

Gracious God, thank You that You do not ask that we be transformed instantly into perfect beings. Only You, O Lord, are perfect. Please help me to develop well-formed maturity as You bring out the best of me through the First Place 4 Health program. Amen.

SQUEEZED INTO THE WORLD'S MOLD

Day 3

Lord, so often I allow the world to dictate how I should think and act. Help me to focus on Christ as the standard for my life. Amen.

Yesterday we examined Eugene Peterson's paraphrase of this week's memory verse. What did you learn from looking at this paraphrase that you might have missed had we not looked at Romans 12:2 in *THE MESSAGE*?

In the Phillips translation, Romans 12:2 is worded like this:

> *Don't let the world around you squeeze you into its own mould, but let God re-make you so that your whole attitude of mind is changed. Thus you will prove in practice that the will of God is good, acceptable to him and perfect.*

According to Phillips, what is the world around us trying to do?

This particular passage has rich application for those of us who have struggled with weight and body image. What mold has the world tried to squeeze you into, and what happened to your genuine God-fashioned self in the process? This can look like anything from striving to mirror fashion models who make up less than one percent of the population and have been airbrushed, touched up and made up by a crew of very talented people to obsessively comparing yourself; to comparing yourself to others instead of to Christ as the highest standard of unfading beauty and attractiveness; to climbing the corporate ladder with little regard for others. Think carefully before you answer!

According to the Phillips translation, God wants to "re-make you so that your whole attitude of mind is changed." How is that statement similar to what we read yesterday in *THE MESSAGE*?

How might this *Begin with Christ* Bible study be part of changing your whole attitude?

The Phillips translation tells us that we are to allow God to re-make our minds so that we can "prove in practice" that God's will is good. How does the First Place 4 Health program prove in practice that God's will is good for you and pleasing to Him?

How does the First Place 4 Health program help you obey God's command to love Him with all your heart, mind, spirit and strength, and care for yourself as a reflection of His great love for you?

How is this obedience to God's commands different from meeting the demands of quick-fix diet and exercise programs that do not stress balance and holistic health?

According to *THE MESSAGE* translation of Romans 12:2 that we studied yesterday, God's desire for us is maturity—"well-formed maturity." What is the maturity being spoken of here? Is it merely getting old, or is it developing all aspects of our being to their full potential? Thoroughly explain your answer, and make it specific to your health and fitness efforts.

What happens when our body ages but we still have the instant-gratification mentality of an immature child?

How is the First Place 4 Health program growing you up in your faith and in your emotions and thoughts?

O merciful Father, forgive me for the times I have squeezed into the world's mold the body You carefully fashioned. Help me to walk in authenticity before You rather than becoming a projection of what the world expects me to be. Amen.

A LESSON FROM A MUSTARD SEED

Day 4

Gracious God, so often I grow impatient. Help me to learn to wait on Your will, Your way and Your time. Amen.

As we have seen in our lessons thus far this week, there is a big difference between the instant gratification mindset of the society we live in and God's good, pleasing and perfect plan for our lives. While Jesus was here on Earth in human form, He gave us some parables, or stories, that help us better understand what it is like to grow in grace and knowledge. Or as J. B. Phillips put it, they help us learn how to put God's perfect plan into practice—to apply Kingdom principles to our everyday, ordinary lives. One of these stories is called the Parable of the Mustard Seed.

Turn to Matthew 13:31-32 in your Bible to read this short teaching story. As you read it, remember that a parable is an earthly story that teaches us a Kingdom truth. What did the unnamed man do with the mustard seed?

What does Jesus tell us about the size of the mustard seed?

What does Jesus tell us happens to the mustard seed when it has been planted and has grown to full maturity?

How is Jesus' parable about the growth of the mustard seed different from the instant-gratification mentality of the world we live in?

How is the germination of a seed planted in the ground similar to God's changing us from the inside out?

Church history tells us that Jesus' brother James was a farmer. In his epistle, James talks about the patience of those who plant seeds. Turn to James 5:7. In this verse, James urges us to be patient until the coming of the Lord. Then James goes on to give an example of a farmer who patiently waits for the earth "to yield its valuable crop." What is the valuable crop you are anticipating through participation in First Place 4 Health, and how is patience part of the First Place 4 Health process?

How is the First Place 4 Health program part of the spiritual growth process that turns a tiny mustard seed into a large plant—a tree big enough for birds to nest in?

What might your mustard-seed-sized faith look like after you complete this *Begin with Christ* Bible study? Be creative in your answer. If you are artistic, you can even draw a picture in your journal rather than write an answer.

Loving Lord, thank You for practical examples that teach me how to put my faith words into practice. Help me to nurture my mustard-seed-sized faith, confident that in time it will yield a valuable crop. Amen.

CLIMBING THE LADDER

Day 5

O Lord God, I will keep my eyes on You, confident that when I am focused on Your goodness and grace, the things of this world will pale in comparison to Your glory. Amen.

Yesterday we studied Jesus' parable about the mustard seed. How did your faith in the First Place 4 Health process grow a bit stronger through that study?

Our personal transformation—our renewal—can also be compared to climbing a ladder. As we begin today's study, stop for a moment and compare climbing a ladder to taking an elevator. Both the ladder and the elevator get you to a higher place. But there are critical differences in how you get there. What are the differences, and how do those differences apply to our lessons about gradual transformation?

Our journey of faith is much like climbing a ladder, one rung at a time, until we reach the top. It takes time and effort to move from one rung to the next! As you learned from the comparison of using an elevator, climbing a ladder is not about pushing a button and waiting for some other force to move you quickly to the top.

Look up the verses that appear on the right-hand side of the ladder below, and write a brief summary of that verse in the middle section of the ladder. Next look at the faith-level descriptions on the left-hand side of the ladder. Circle the faith-level you are at right now.

Peaceful faith		Galatians 2:20
Total surrender		Romans 12:1-2
Hunger for righteousness		Matthew 5:6
Partial surrender		Luke 9:57-62
Struggling		Romans 7:19-20
Seeking		Isaiah 55:6-7
Unstable faith		James 1:8

What energy and effort will it take for you to move up to the next rung on your personal-faith ladder?

How might the world's mentality be holding you back, keeping you from advancing in spiritual maturity?

How is that mentality something that hinders and sin that easily entangles us?

O Lord, how thankful I am that You are patient with me as I progress in my faith. Thank You for the promise that You will bring to completion the good work You have begun in me. Amen.

REFLECTION AND APPLICATION

Day 6

Father, Your Word shows me how to live and what You ask of me. Thank You for renewing my mind through the power of Your Word. Amen.

This week we have examined our memory verse as translated in three different Bibles: the *New International Version, THE MESSAGE* and *The New Testament in Modern English*. The *New Living Translation* offers us another interpretation:

> *Don't copy the behavior and customs of this world, but let God transform you into a new person by changing the way you think. Then you will learn to know God's will for you, which is good and pleasing and perfect* (Romans 12:2).

As we begin today's time of reflection and application, think about the world's behaviors and customs as they apply to the quick-fix, instant makeover schemes that appeal to those who need to lose weight—whether it be 20 or 200 pounds. In the left-hand column in the chart below, list five of those programs; and in the right-hand column, tell how they are different from First Place 4 Health. Include medical-solution programs, like surgery, in your list, along with frivolous diets like eating nothing but cabbage soup. There are many programs out there, so try to pick five programs that are representative of the many quick-fix solutions on the market. In the middle column, indicate whether or not you have tried this program and, if so, tell the results of your instant-solution efforts.

World's Quick-Fix Programs	My Experience	First Place 4 Health

Lord God Almighty, those who trust in You and Your ways are never disappointed. Thank You for being the God that I can always rely on and trust. Amen.

REFLECTION AND APPLICATION

Day 7

O gracious God, thank You for the many ways You give me to express my thoughts and feelings. Help me to be creative in my praise and worship of You. Amen.

During our Day Two study, we looked at *THE MESSAGE* translation of our memory verse for the week. In that version of the Bible, the last part of Romans 12:2 reads, "Unlike the culture around you, always dragging you down to its level of immaturity, God brings the best out of you, develops well-formed maturity in you."

Today during your reflection and application time, take two pieces of blank paper. At the top of one page, write, "Dragging Me Down." At the top of the other, write, "Bringing the Best Out of Me." Then on each piece of paper, describe what those words look like in practical terms with regard to eating.

You can draw pictures if you are artistic, do a mind map if you are a logical thinker, or make a collage of pictures cut from magazines if you are visually oriented. If you are musical, on one sheet you might want to write the words of a song that describes being dragged down, and on the other sheet, the words of a song that epitomizes being built up. Be creative with this exercise as God uses it to transform you from the inside out. Share your descriptions with your First Place 4 Health group this week.

Lord God Almighty, there is such a difference between the way You treat me and what the world does to me as it tries to squeeze me into its mold. Thank You for the freedom I have in Jesus Christ my Lord. Amen.

Group Prayer Requests

first place 4 health

Today's Date: ____________________

Name	Request

Results

____

____

____

____

____

____

____

Week Nine

filled with the Spirit

Scripture Memory Verse

Do you not know that your body is a temple of the Holy Spirit, who is in you, whom you have received from God? You are not your own; you were bought at a price. Therefore honor God with your body.

1 Corinthians 6:19-20

Although this renewal process we call sanctification takes a lifetime, there is one thing in God's kingdom that is instantaneous! The very moment we confess Jesus as our Lord and Savior, the Spirit of the living Lord, God's Holy Spirit, takes up residence in our heart—not as an honored guest, but as the One sent from God to come alongside us, direct our path and lead us into all truth. The apostle Paul, in this week's memory verse, urges us to remember that our body has become the Spirit's temple, the Spirit's dwelling place, and we are to care for our body in a way that honors the Spirit who dwells within.

The word "therefore" at the beginning of the last sentence in our memory verse invites us to look back at the previous statement in order to properly understand the second. Why are we to honor God with our body?

What was the price "you were bought at," and who paid it?

If you lived in moment-by-moment awareness that the Spirit lives in your heart by faith, how might that impact your First Place 4 Health program, especially as it applies to the type of food you put into the Spirit's temple, and why?

Day 1

GUEST BENEFITS

Gracious God, it is beyond my comprehension that the Spirit of the living Lord would live in my humble heart! Help me to honor You in all I say and do. Amen.

When we make reservations to stay in a hotel, one of the first things we look at is the amenities, the guest benefits we will receive for staying in the place. But in God's kingdom, the Spirit does not consider the benefits He will receive when He takes up residence in our heart. Rather, He offers *us* benefits! Just before Jesus was crucified, He told His grieving disciples about some of the benefits the Holy Spirit would bring. Turn to John 14:15-21 in your Bible.

Before we begin to examine this passage, do you recognize John 14:21? If so, where have you seen it before?

Yes, John 14:21 was our Week Four memory verse! What is promised in this verse if we obey Jesus' commands?

According to John 14:21, what does our obedience prove, and how is this like what J. B. Phillips, in last week's study, called "proving by practice"?

Now look at John 14:15. What does this verse tell us about our love for Jesus?

In John 14:16, we are told about another benefit of being obedient to Jesus' commands. What will Jesus ask the Father to give those who obey God's commands?

How long will this gift be with us (see John 14:16)?

How is something that lasts forever different from instant gratification?

Verse 17 gives us the name of the gift that the Father will send at Jesus' request. What is the gift, and why can't the world accept this gift from the Father?

How do we know the Spirit, and how does John 14:17 affirm this week's memory verse?

According to John 14:18, Jesus promised not to leave His frightened disciples "as orphans." Instead, He promised to come to them. In verse 17, the Spirit of truth was identified as the One sent. How are Jesus and the Spirit of truth one and the same person?

If someone unfamiliar with the Bible were to ask you to show them an example of the Trinity in Scripture, how could you use John 14:15-21 to show the interaction of the Father, the Son and the Holy Spirit?

According to verse 19, Jesus told His disciples:

Because I ____________, you also will ____________.

Recall the three types of life discussed during Week Seven. Which life do you think Jesus is speaking of in this verse, and why?

O Lord, thank You that You have not left me a spiritual orphan. In love and compassion You sent the Holy Spirit to be with me forever. How can I ever express my gratitude for Your mercy, compassion and love? Amen.

Day 2

THE SPIRIT OF TRUTH

O Lord, You are faithful and You are loving. Help me to understand the truth You want to impart to me today through this Bible study lesson. Amen.

Yesterday we began to look at the many benefits that are ours because the Spirit of the living Lord has taken up residence in our humble heart. What did you learn from yesterday's lesson that will help you live in the constant awareness that your body is the Spirit's home?

According to John 14:24-25, Jesus talked about where the words He has given His followers came from. What was the source of everything Jesus said?

Although Jesus was faithful to speak the words His Father gave Him, the disciples were often slow learners. They quickly forgot what Jesus told them, often falling back into old habits. But they were not without hope. Who would be with them forever and continually remind them of what Jesus taught them while He was still here on Earth?

What does the use of the words "all" and "everything" in verse John 14:26 tell you?

How does the Holy Spirit guide us into all truth (see John 14:26)?

What has the Holy Spirit taught you during this *Begin with Christ* Bible study? Has He reminded you of portions of God's Word you have heard before? What else has He taught you that will help you in your First Place 4 Health efforts?

John 14:30 tells us that someone is about to interrupt Jesus' teaching, someone called "the prince of this world." Recall from your earlier studies who this prince of the world is. How is the prince of the world different from the Holy Spirit Jesus sent to His disciples?

During Day Seven last week, we spent time illustrating two realities about eating: One was the things of this world that drag us down; the other was the best that God brings out of us. How is the prince of the world one of the things that drag us down, and how is God's Spirit the One who brings out our best?

Jesus said that the prince of the world has no hold on Him (see John 14:30). Why do you think that statement is true?

Even though Satan has no hold on Jesus, Jesus allowed Himself to be taken away for a specific reason. Read John 14:31, and write down what you learn.

How is all of this part of the price you were bought at, and what are we to do because Jesus was obedient to the Father, even to death?

O Jesus, You were obedient to the Father, even when obedience was painful. Help me, through the power of Your Spirit, to do exactly what You ask me to do. Amen.

ALWAYS WITH US

Day 3

O Lord, You have promised to never leave me or forsake me. Thank You for being close to me when I am sick, sad, lonely or grieving. Amen.

In John 11, we are told about the death of Lazarus, the brother of Mary and Martha. Jesus was a guest in their home in Bethany on several occasions. What does John 11:5 tell us about the relationship Jesus shared with Mary, Martha and Lazarus?

Even though Jesus loved Lazarus, when Mary and Martha's brother got very sick, Jesus was many miles away and couldn't help. In His physical body, Jesus had the same limitations we have; He could not be in two places at one time. Lazarus's sickness ended in death. When Jesus finally got to Judea, what was the first thing Martha said to Jesus (see John 11:21)?

Jesus was not physically present to heal Lazarus, and He was not there to comfort the sisters as their brother was dying. Later, Jesus would turn this tragedy into a miracle and teach the mourners a powerful "I Am" lesson—He is the Resurrection, the Truth and the Life—when He called Lazarus out of the tomb, much like He calls us out of our spiritual darkness into His marvelous light.

Turn to John 16:7 in your Bible. Jesus' disciples were filled with grief because Jesus was going to leave them, but Jesus told them that His departure was for their benefit. What was the truth Jesus taught them?

When Jesus took up residence in the disciples' heart as the Spirit of the resurrected Lord, He would always be with them. There would never come a time in the life of Jesus' followers when He would not be with them!

According to John 16:11, what will happen to the prince of this world when the Spirit comes?

According to John 16:12, Jesus clearly told His disciples that He had a lot more to teach them, but they were not ready to hear what He had to say. According to verses 13-14, who is it that will take up where Jesus left off, and what will that Person do? Explain what John 16:13-14 teaches in your own words.

According to John 16:33, why did Jesus take the time to explain all this to His disciples?

What did Jesus tell us we will have in this world?

How is the prince of this world part of the trouble we will experience while we are living here on Earth?

What has Jesus done on our behalf?

Spend time praising Jesus that He has overcome the world and promised that those who believe in Him will do the same!

O merciful Lord, I am encouraged by Your words, "Take heart." Even in Your own agony, You took the time to reassure Your disciples, and through them You encourage my heart, too. Amen.

PRAYING IN THE SPIRIT

Day 4

Thank You, Lord God, that You know my weakness and hear my prayers through the power of the Holy Spirit. Amen.

After Jesus had ascended into heaven to take His rightful place at the right hand of the Father, Jesus' followers experienced the power from on high. As they were praying in the Upper Room, a mighty wind came and tongues of fire descended on them. The Spirit had indeed come. That was the first Pentecost, the day the timid disciples became bold witnesses for the risen Lord. As the days and months and years went by, Jesus' faithful followers learned more and more about this wonderful gift called the Holy Spirit.

The apostle Paul, in Romans 8:26-27, tells us about a benefit we receive from the Spirit's presence that is very important to our efforts in First Place 4 Health. Turn to Romans 8 in your Bible, and read Paul's words. Paul begins by telling us, "The Spirit helps us in our weakness." Recall the inventory you did at the beginning of this study. What were your weaknesses, and what is the Spirit available to do for you?

Not only will the Spirit help us by bringing Jesus' teaching to mind (which we learned about earlier this week), but also the Spirit does something else. In Romans 8:26, what does Paul tell us the Spirit does for us?

Does the fact that we don't know what to pray for, or even how to pray, limit our ability to come to the Lord in our time of need? Why or why not?

Recall a time when you were so burdened with grief and cares that you could not even begin to express what was going on inside you. According to Romans 8:26, who is able to interpret your sighs and times of intense sadness or uncertainty?

Having interpreted those inner feelings you could not describe, much less express, what does the Spirit then do?

At the conclusion of Romans 8:27, Paul tells us:

The Spirit ______ for the ______ in ______ with God's ______.

Who else is sitting at the right hand of the Father, interceding for us? (Refer to Hebrews 4:14-16 if you are not sure of the answer.)

Jesus, the great high priest, is interceding for you. The Spirit is interceding for you, too. Yes, *you!* All who believe in the Lord Jesus Christ are considered saints in the New Testament. There is a great cloud of witnesses cheering you on, both by example and through the written word of God. Explain how all these benefits allow you to run the First Place 4 Health race and overcome the things that threaten to throw you off course!

Now read 2 Timothy 1:7. What do we learn about the Spirit God has given us?

How are love, power and self-discipline part of the benefits you enjoy because the Holy Spirit has taken up residence in your heart-home? Give concrete examples.

Is the Spirit pleased when we ignore all these wonderful benefits and try to achieve our health and fitness goals in our own strength and power? Why or why not?

Forgive me, living Lord, when I shrink back in fear rather than realize that the Spirit You give me brings love and power and self-discipline, even as He intercedes for me in a language I do not understand. Amen.

FILLED WITH THE SPIRIT

Day 5

My Lord and my God, at times it would be easier to ignore Your words than put them into practice. Help me to be faithful to my First Place 4 Health commitment, even when to do so is difficult. Amen.

Although we try hard to separate different forms of self-indulgence into neat little categories—alcoholics in one box, overeaters in another, compulsive spend-ers in yet another, worriers in another, and sex addicts in a category all by themselves—God does not. Scripture is very clear that any form of self-indulgent excess is an affront to God. Yes, in the physical realm the consequences may be different, but in God's eyes, anything that fills the space where His Spirit longs to dwell is sinful. Turn to Proverbs 23:19-21, and summarize in your own words what you learn.

How is your willingness to go along with other overeaters different from your willingness to party with alcoholics? Why?

Proverbs 23:19-21 tells us that all forms of excess make us poor. What type of poverty is the proverb speaking of?

According to Proverbs 19:21, in addition to suffering spiritual poverty, indulgers in the sin of excess also experience "____________ [which] clothes them in ____________." Give an example of how this proverb applied to your life before coming to First Place 4 Health. (Remember that "drowsiness" and "rags" are used here both symbolically and literally.)

In Ephesians 5:17-18, at the beginning of verse 17, Paul tells us not to "be foolish." Drawing on all you have learned in the *Begin with Christ* Bible study so far, how is indulging in any form of excess foolish?

Ephesians 5:17 exhorts us to "understand what the Lord's will is." From our earlier studies, when we conform to the standards of this world, can we discern God's will? Explain your answer.

In Ephesians 5:18, Paul issues a very strong command. What does Paul tell us not to do, and why?

What do you think the word "debauchery" means?

Look up the word "debauchery" in a dictionary. What did you discover? (You will probably find two meanings given. Write them both down.)

When we engage in excess, we harm ourselves and we lead others astray. How do you lead others astray when you do not control your own appetite?

Instead of engaging in excess, what luxury does the apostle Paul tell us to indulge in (see Ephesians 5:18)?

Excess leads to debauchery, but what does being filled with the Spirit lead to?

Ephesians 5:19-20 gives us the wonderful alternative to causing harm to self and leading others astray. How is singing psalms and hymns and spiritual songs part of your First Place 4 Health lifestyle?

What about giving thanks for everything? Do you make it a consistent practice to give thanks to God at all times and in all circumstances? If not, why not?

In First Place 4 Health, we encourage our fellow health-and-fitness companions. How does Ephesians 5:19-20 encourage us to encourage others?

Spend the rest of your study time today praising God, as you are filled with the Spirit. And while you are filled with God's abundance, send a word of encouragement to someone in your First Place 4 Health group who is struggling with excess right now.

O Lord God, forgive me for those times I indulge my physical appetites rather than allow You to lavish me with Your love. Thank You, Father, for forgiveness and the opportunity to be filled with the Spirit! Amen.

Day 6

REFLECTION AND APPLICATION

O Lord Christ, You came so that I might experience joy and peace and contentment. Forgive me for those times I settle for the little kingdom of this world rather than seek Your kingdom and a right relationship with You. Amen.

Throughout our *Begin with Christ* Bible study, we have learned that there are two powerful leaders at work in the world. Who are these two leaders?

Both of these powerful rulers have a kingdom. Jesus called Satan the prince of this world. The other kingdom is the kingdom of God. What did you learn about the kingdom of God in our Week Two memory verse?

But the kingdom of the prince of this world is very different. Remember that John 10:10 tells us that the devil is the one who kills, destroys and steals. And while God's kingdom is full of the abundant life, Satan's kingdom might well be called the "Kingdom of the Littles":

Little self-control
Little discipline
Little obedience
Little sacrifice
Little accountability
Little responsibility
Little patience

LEAD TO

Little blessing
Little freedom
Little contentment
Little unity
Little joy
Little faith
Little hope

As you look over this list, in each group pick one of the Littles that you are experiencing in your life right now, even though you are filled with the Spirit of love, power and self-control. Circle the two problem areas you identify. Next, see if you can find a correlation between the two Littles you have circled. For instance, what might the correlation be between "Little discipline" and "Little joy"? You will need to give this exercise careful thought; most of all you will need to be searchingly honest about the condition of your life in Christ. List your problem Littles in your spiritual journal, and write about the correlation between each problem and what it leads to.

Heavenly Father, thank You for sending Jesus to rescue me from the Kingdom of the Littles and bring me into the Kingdom of Your lavish light and love. Amen.

Day 7

REFLECTION AND APPLICATION

Thank You, gracious God, for the gift of song and for words and music that allow me to worship You in spirit and in truth. Amen.

This week we have learned about just a few of the many, many benefits that are ours because the Holy Spirit has taken up residence in our heart. During our Day Five study, we learned that we are to "sing and make music" in our heart to God. Today, rather than writing, we are going to follow the apostle Paul's command and sing our praise and thanksgiving to the God who loves us and gave His Son for us.

Think of a favorite hymn or praise song you would like to use in your serenade to God today. Remember that how well you sing is not important; it is that you are willing to obediently sing His praises that pleases God. When we sing our praises to God on high, we can truly sing like there's nobody listening—no one, that is, except the One who loves to hear us sing, even when we are off-key.

Our voice in song is music to our Father's ears! It is our joyful noise that pleases Him! Spend your devotion time today singing God's praises, and then carry that wonderful melody with you throughout your day!

It is good to sing praise to Your name, O Lord, Most High. Amen.

Group Prayer Requests

Today's Date: ____________________

Name	Request

Results

____

____

____

____

____

____

____

Week Ten

more commitment

Scripture Memory Verse

Commit to the Lord whatever you do,
and your plans will succeed.

Proverbs 16:3

Scripture is very specific. There are two kingdoms, two moral codes, two sets of values and two very different rulers who contend for our loyalty. One kingdom is ruled by the prince of this world. It is characterized by darkness and deception, discord, destruction and lies. The other kingdom, God's kingdom, is characterized by light and revelation, love, commitment and truth. As we have seen throughout the *Begin with Christ* Bible study, at each juncture in the road, we have a choice. We can either choose to seek God's kingdom and reap the rewards of being in a right relationship with the sovereign Lord of heaven and Earth, or we can bow down and worship the prince of this world as we allow ourselves to be squeezed into the world's dark, oppressive mold. We can choose either to be part of the Kingdom of the Littles or to live the abundant life the Good Shepherd came to give those who hear His voice and obey His commands. We can choose life, or we can choose destruction.

First Place 4 Health is founded on God's life-giving Word. Pause for a few moments as we begin this week's study, and think about the life-affirming choices you have made in the past eight weeks as a direct result of what you have learned during this First Place 4 Health session. What is the most significant change you have made, and what has been the positive result of that change?

COMMITMENT BREAKS THE WORLD'S MOLD

Day 1

O Lord God, there is no freedom outside of a committed relationship with You. Thank You for being faithful to me. Help me to be faithful to You, too. Amen.

Our Week Eight memory verse warned us not to ______ to the patterns of this world, but instead be ______ by the ______ of our ______. Summarize what you learned during the Week Eight lessons about the dangers of being squeezed into the world's mold.

And as we think about all the ways in which the world's mindset keeps us struggling with sin rather than cooperating with God as He works to bring the best out of us, very few of us would list *commitment* as a virtue. We have been so influenced by the commitment-phobic society we live in that the very word has taken on a negative connotation for most of us. "Keep your options open" is the message the world continually touts. Keep your options open, because commitment is a trap that will keep you from doing what pleases you at the moment. But as our memory verse for this week tells us, in God's kingdom, commitment is not only a virtue, but it is also the pathway to success.

Write this week's memory verse, then circle the words "commit to the Lord."

What is the first commitment we are to make to our Lord and Savior, Jesus Christ, and why is that to be our number one priority? (Hint: The answer is found in our Week Two memory verse.)

When you joined First Place 4 Health, you also made another commitment. What was that commitment, and to whom did you commit those plans ? (You made a commitment to two people, so list them both!)

Have you been faithful to the commitment you made before beginning this First Place 4 Health session to God and to yourself? List the ways in which you have honored your commitment to health and balance.

From what you learned during our Week Eight study about the transformation process, why is it important that you commit to the First Place 4 Health program for one year rather than think attendance at one session is enough? Explain your answer thoroughly.

How is making a commitment to First Place 4 Health different from keeping your options open and looking for other alternatives as you halfheartedly go through the motions of doing the First Place 4 Health program?

Have you made that one-year commitment to health and fitness? Why or why not?

O Lord God, thank You for Your faithfulness and love. You have made a commitment to never leave me or forsake me, and You have been true to Your Word. Help me to honor my commitment to You, too. Amen.

Day 2

GOD'S COMMITMENT TO YOU

O Lord, You are faithful and true to all You promise.
Those who trust in You are never disappointed. Amen.

Write out our memory verse again today. Then highlight (or underline) the word "commit."

Look up the word "commit" in a dictionary, and list the meanings you find.

What new thing(s) did you learn about the word "commit" from the definitions?

"Commit" comes from two Latin words that together essentially mean "to send, as on a mission." What two missions, or purposes, do we bring together when we commit our plans to the Lord?

Commitment brings us in line with God's will. We commit to doing things His way and in sync with His will rather than stubbornly trying to do things our way and asking Him to bless our misguided efforts.

One of the wonderful things about our God is that He never asks us to do anything for Him that He has not first done for us! So in considering our commitment to God, we need to always be mindful of His everlasting commitment to us. When the Israelites were about to be led out of the cruel slavery of Egypt, God appeared to Moses and made a commitment to His Chosen People.

Turn to Exodus 6:6-8 in your Bible, and after reading the passage, list the four commitments God made to His people.

First, God promised to free His people from the yoke of slavery. How has God, through your participation in the First Place 4 Health program, freed you from the bondage of compulsive overeating?

Second, God promised to redeem His people "with an outstretched arm and with mighty acts." How has God's commitment to stretch out His arm and do mighty things been part of your salvation story? You might want to picture Jesus' outstretched arms on that cross at Calvary as you contemplate your answer.

Next, God promised to take the Israelites as His people and to be their God. How has God been faithful to His commitment to be your loving Lord and Master, to make you part of His family and to love you as a precious child?

Finally, God promised to give His people the land He covenanted to give Abraham—the Promised Land. This is a promise that God fulfilled in part when Joshua led God's people across the Jordan River; however, it has yet to be completely fulfilled. What is the Promised Land we are still waiting to inherit?

God keeps His promises! He is a God of commitment who expects His people to make a commitment to Him, too. What promise of God do you need to cling to as you move forward toward your Promised Land?

O Lord, Your mercies are new every morning, and Your faithfulness is great. Thank You for showing me how to live out my commitment to keep You first in all things. Amen.

ACCOUNTABILITY REINFORCES COMMITMENT

Day 3

O God, when I consider what You have done for me, I am humbled.
When I consider what I have done for You, I am ashamed.
Please forgive me for not being as committed to You as You are to me. Amen.

"Accountability," like "commitment," is not a word the society we live in values or affirms. Yet in God's kingdom, accountability and commitment go together like a hand and a glove. When we make a commitment to God and to ourselves, we need to also make that commitment to a group of others who will hold us accountable to our words. How has your First Place 4 Health group been your accountability partners during this segment of your journey to health and wholeness? In answering this question, remember that accountability partners do not flatter with false compliments or affirm the things we are doing wrong!

While we may erroneously think of accountability as a negative thing, King Solomon, the wisest of the wise, listed the benefits of having people to hold us up. Turn to Ecclesiastes 4:9-12, and read the list. What is the first benefit Solomon lists in verse 9?

How has your First Place 4 Health group been part of the good return you have gotten from your health and fitness efforts through the First Place 4 Health program?

What dimension would your good efforts have lacked if you were making this journey alone?

Ecclesiastes 4:10 mentions an ever-present reality of our human condition: No matter how stable we think we may be, there will be times when we will fall. What happens to someone who falls and does not have anyone to help him or her get up again?

Think of a time during this First Place 4 Health session when you have "fallen." Who was there to help you up, and what did this person do to help you get back on track?

Read Ecclesiastes 4:11. How has your First Place 4 Health group been a source of warmth for you? Describe what that warmth felt like. Was it mental, emotional, physical or spiritual? How did it help you remain faithful to the commitment you have made to health and wholeness?

Ecclesiastes 4:12 tells us that two can better defend themselves; two can stand firm rather than being overpowered. How has your First Place 4 Health group been a source of strength to you, part of the way out God has provided for you when you were being tempted?

Carefully read the last sentence of verse 12. Suddenly the two have become a cord of three strands. Who is the third person in the cord, and how is this person the One who binds the other two together?

End your time today by writing a note of gratitude to one of the people in your First Place 4 Health group who has helped you remain faithful to your commitment to honor your body because of God's great commitment to you.

O Lord God, You provide for all my needs. At a time when I felt isolated and alone, You brought me into the loving fellowship of First Place 4 Health. Thank You! Amen.

COMMIT AND SERVE

Day 4

O Lord, You are my strength and my shield.
You are the One who delivers me when I humble myself
and return to You with all my heart. Amen.

Samuel was committed to the Lord by his mother long before his conception and birth. So when Samuel was a young boy, his mother, Hannah, took him to Eli the priest, in keeping with her vow to the Lord. From that day forward, Samuel faithfully served the Lord and ministered to God's people by bringing the word of the Lord to them. When the Ark of the Lord had been stolen away by Israel's enemies, the Philistines, the people of Israel mourned and sought after the Lord. In response to their cries for help, God sent Samuel the prophet to speak to them on His behalf. Turn now to 1 Samuel 7:3 in your Bible. Samuel said to God's grieving people that day:

> If you are ________________ to the ____________ with ________ your ____________, then ______________ yourselves of the foreign ____________ and the Ashtoreths and ____________ yourselves to the ____________ and ______________ him only, and he will ______________ you out of the hand of the Philistines.

How do Samuel's words correspond with the words of our Week Ten memory verse?

____

____

____

First Samuel 7:2 tells us that the Ark of the Lord, containing the Ten Commandments and symbolizing God's Word and covenant promises, had been absent for 20 years. The people to whom Samuel spoke God's words had a desire to return to the Lord. They wanted to enjoy God's protection and provision. They were tired of chasing after foreign gods and reaping the consequences of disobedience.

Many of us come to First Place 4 Health because, like the Israelites, we want to return to the Lord after a long time of living in disobedience and despair when it comes to self-care. Do you have a "time away from God" story? If so, be detailed in your explanation. Write about how long you wandered in disobedience with regard to health and fitness, and list the consequences you have suffered because of your estrangement from God's will and way. If you prefer, record your answer in your spiritual journal.

____

____

____

____

____

Samuel's words to the Israelites that day were what we call an "if-then" statement. An "if-then" statement is one in which the "then" only happens once the "if" has been fulfilled. Look carefully at the words of 1 Samuel 7:3. What is the "if" the Israelites would need to fulfill in order for the "then" to become reality? What would be the "then"?

What do the words "with all your hearts" signify?

Samuel told the people to rid themselves of their foreign gods and their pagan symbols so that they could fully commit themselves to the Lord. How is this like throwing off all the things that hinder and entangle us?

If the Israelites had not gotten rid of the foreign gods and pagan symbols, would God have kept His promise to deliver them out of the hands of the Philistines?

The Philistines may have been a race of giant people. What giants are you facing in your life when it comes to health, balance and wholeness? How can you apply Samuel's words to your present situation?

How are you being asked to make a commitment and serve the Lord your God through the First Place 4 Health program?

O Lord God, You have promised to redeem me from my painful past when I am willing to put away all the false gods I have served and when I return to You with all my heart. Thank You for Your compassion and love. Amen.

Day 5

COMMITMENT CONTINUES TO DO GOOD

O God, there will be times when I suffer because I have made a commitment to do Your will. Jesus, my leader and example, suffered, too. Just as Jesus focused on the joy set before Him, I need to see the joy set before me as I am faithful to my commitment to You. Please help me. Amen.

The apostle Peter knew firsthand the consequences of making a commitment to the Lord and then failing to keep that vow. On the night before Jesus was crucified, Peter made a bold commitment. Turn to Mark 14:27-31 in your Bible. What did Peter emphatically vow to do?

But hours later, Jesus' prediction became a reality. Turn to Mark 14:66-72. What happened to Peter's commitment to stand by his Lord, no matter what?

Years later, Peter taught others the lesson he learned through that painful experience. Turn to 1 Peter 4:19. In your own words, as if you were teaching someone else, write what Peter taught.

What does "suffer according to God's will" mean? Does it mean to suffer because we have made a commitment to uphold God's will, no matter what, or does it mean it is God's will that we suffer? Explain your answer!

How does Peter's statement here correspond to Jesus' statement recorded in John 16:33, which tells us that in this world we will have trouble?

How have you suffered according to God's will because of your commitment to the First Place 4 Health program? What does this tell you about the cost of commitment?

First Place 4:19 also tells us that we are to ________ ourselves to our ________ ________. What type of commitment is Peter talking about? (Before answering this question, you might want to refer back to our discussion of commitment in this week's Day One study.)

And in addition to allowing our faithful Creator to right the wrongs being done to us because we are faithful to His Word and way, what else does 1 Peter 4:19 tell us to do?

________ to do ________.

Think back to some of the ways you have suffered because of your commitment to First Place 4 Health. How were you able to continue to do good in the face of opposition?

The apostle Paul, a man who suffered greatly for his commitment to Jesus Christ, told us what to do when we find ourselves being afflicted because of our commitment to God. Turn to Romans 12:21. What did Paul say, and how can you apply his words to your First Place 4 Health program?

Gracious God, how thankful I am for Your Word. When I am in need of comfort, all I need to do is turn to the pages of Scripture and renew my commitment to You. Amen.

Day 6

REFLECTION AND APPLICATION

Gracious Lord, when I fix my eyes on You and not on the cares of this world, I am able to fulfill my commitment to give You first place in my life. Amen.

We are nearing the end of our *Begin with Christ* Bible study, with only one more week of lessons to complete before finishing this leg of the lifelong journey we are making toward health, wholeness and a lifestyle that honors God, our Creator. This is an excellent time to review what we have done in the past nine weeks. You have memorized nine Scripture verses and learned many new ways to apply those verses to your First Place 4 Health endeavors. Write the memory verse for each week; then summarize how you have been able to apply that verse, and the lesson it reinforced, to your new life-giving lifestyle.

Week Two:

Week Three:

Week Four:

Week Five:

Week Six:

Week Seven:

Week Eight:

Week Nine:

Week Ten:

Spend the rest of your reflection and application time praising God for the marvelous ways He has transformed your life because you have made a commitment to love and serve Him with all your heart.

Almighty and merciful Father, today I will praise You, for You have been good to me. You have been faithful to Your promises and Your word. Help me to honor my commitments to You, myself and my First Place 4 Health companions. Amen.

Day 7

REFLECTION AND APPLICATION

Thank You, gracious Lord, that You have promised to bring to completion the good work You have begun in me. Amen.

As we draw near to the close of this session of First Place 4 Health, it is important that we remember the words of this week's memory verse and continue to commit our plans to the Lord. What are your health and fitness goals, and how will First Place 4 Health be a part of those plans during the months and years ahead? Spend some time today committing yourself to the plans God has for you. Remember that He is the One bringing out the best of you. He is working all things together for His glory and for your good. He has committed to bring the good work He began in you to completion, but you must be willing to do your part, too. Write down your hopes and dreams, and discuss how First Place 4 Health will be part of the good things God has in store for you in the future. Remember that God has given you the Holy Spirit to lead you into all truth. By making prayer part of your planning, you will be committing your plans to God so that they will succeed.

Thank You, loving Lord, for sending the Holy Spirit to be my counselor and guide. When I commit my plans to You and walk in sync with the Spirit, my life will bring glory and honor to You. Amen.

Group Prayer Requests

first place 4 health

Today's Date: ____________

Name	Request

Results

Week Eleven

love defines discipleship

Scripture Memory Verse

A new command I give you: Love one another. As I have loved you, so you must love one another. By this all men will know that you are my disciples, if you love one another.

John 13:34-35

Jesus Christ, the Word of God in human flesh, came to Earth to show us the love of the Father. Throughout the Old Testament, God told His people how much He loved them. He protected them, provided for them, prospered them and planted them in a land flowing with milk and honey. Yet in spite of God's words and actions, God's Chosen People continued to rebel against Him and disregard His Word. God sent prophets to preach reform, and the people stoned and killed them. Finally, God sent His own Son to Earth as a sign of His great love for His people. The apostle John described it this way: "The Word became flesh and made his dwelling among us. We have seen his glory, the glory of the One and Only, who came from the Father, full of grace and truth" (John 1:14).

In the first week of the *Begin with Christ* Bible study, we made getting to know more about Jesus, the One we strive to put first in all things, one of our goals. Faith is not foolishness, and to put our trust in someone or something we don't know to be trustworthy is an instant replay of our past, not part of the new behavior that honors God. After 10 weeks of concentrated Bible study, what have you learned about Jesus that convinces you He is deserving of your trust—and of the first place in your life?

HOW MUCH DO YOU LOVE ME?

Day 1

Lord God, forgive me for the times I have tested Your love rather than accepting it as a precious gift. Amen.

"How much do you love me?" the child playfully asks the parent, knowing what the reply will be. And in a delightful and anticipated response, the parent stretches out his or her arms as far as he or she can stretch and replies, "I love you *this* much!"

Long after the childhood years have given way to adulthood, most of us are still asking that same question of the important people in our life: "How much do you love me?" Sometimes the question is direct and playful, like the child's question. But at other times, it is veiled and subtle, characteristic of what psychologists call *passive aggression*. Instead of asking a question, we engage in unacceptable behavior as a way of getting people to affirm that they love us, warts and all.

Many of us play those same passive aggressive games with God, testing His love and asking that He protect and provide for us even when our behavior is anything but loving. Recall from Day Three of your Week Six study how Jesus replied to the devil when our Savior was asked to put God to the test. What did Jesus do, and what did Jesus say? (You may refer back to the earlier lesson or look at Matthew 4:7 if you don't remember the answer.)

How have you tested God's love for you when it comes to caring for the marvelous body He fashioned and entrusted to your care? Be specific in your answer.

Turn to John 3:16-17 in your Bible. How much does God love you? Write God's answer as it appears in your Bible, except *personalize it* by writing your name instead of "the world" in the text.

So often we think of God as a punitive parent, just waiting for us to give Him just cause to scold and punish us. Instead, what truth is found in John 3:17?

If Jesus did not come to Earth to condemn you, what was His reason for coming to Earth in human form?

Paul, writing to the Christians in Rome, answered the "how much does God love us" question from a different perspective. Turn to Romans 8:31-32. Paul, in typical rabbinical teaching fashion, answers our "how much does God love us" question with a question of his own. Rephrase Paul's statement in your own words, changing it from a question to a bold affirmation of faith in God's love.

Lest we think we did anything to deserve God's love, Romans 5:8 tells us what we were like when Jesus died for us, and what His death demonstrated. What was our condition when Christ died for us?

How would you like to respond to God for His great love for you? Remember, God showed His love in a very practical, tangible way, so make your response practical and tangible, too. (John 14:21, our Week Four memory verse, might help you formulate your answer.)

O Lord, all my loving words are of no value if I do not back them up with joyful obedience. Thank You for sending Jesus to show me what real love looks like. Amen.

GOD'S LOVE AND OURS

Day 2

O sovereign Lord, it is impossible for me to comprehend the height and depth, breadth and width of Your love. My finite mind cannot even begin to comprehend what perfect love looks like. Help me, O God, to learn how to love You in increasing measure as I grow in grace and knowledge of the Lord Jesus Christ. Amen.

Our Week Eleven memory verse comes from the Gospel of John. Write out the memory verse. Then circle the words "love" and "loved."

Although we would use the word "loved" to indicate a love that took place in the past, a more correct translation of what Jesus said is that God is perpetually loving. He loved us, He loves us and He will continue to love us throughout eternity. How has God demonstrated His love for you in the past?

How does God demonstrate His love for you in the present moment?

How will God continue to love you even after you are no longer living here on Earth?

How is your participation in the First Place 4 Health program a manifestation of God's love—past, present and future?

How can First Place 4 Health become a perpetual expression of your love for God—past, present and future?

Although God's love for us is perfect, ours for Him is being perfected day by day as we listen to His voice and obey His commands. How will you be able to express your love for God more and more as you grow in grace and knowledge of our Lord Jesus Christ?

Last week, our lessons focused on commitment. How do love and commitment go hand in hand? Can you have one without the other? Why or why not?

What does your commitment in action through faithful adherence to the First Place 4 Health program say about your love for Jesus Christ?

O Lord, it is easy to say I love You, but it is much harder to give practical expression to those words. When I commit myself to doing things Your way, I am agreeing to bring my will under Your authority. Amen.

LOVING WORLDLY THINGS

Day 3

O Lord, there is no way I can love You and love the things of this world. My actions, not my words, declare where my loyalties lie. Help me, gracious God, to choose wisely. Amen.

Our memory verse for this week comes from the Gospel written by John, the one who is often called the "beloved disciple." In order to see how John got that description, turn to John 21:20. Remember, John is the writer of this account, so what do John's words tell you about "the disciple whom Jesus loved"?

If you were writing this account, could you also describe yourself as the "disciple whom Jesus loved"? Why or why not?

In addition to writing the Gospel of John, the apostle John wrote three short letters to the early Christians; and he also wrote the book of Revelation, a vivid description of a vision he received directly from God. In our Week Five study, we looked at John's words about the "lust of [sinful people's] eyes" (1 John 2:16). What do you recall about the people in that study who allowed the lust of their eyes to lead them into sin?

But the lust of the eyes isn't the only thing John addressed in that passage. Turn to 1 John 2:15-17. What is the first thing John tells us in these verses?

Do not ________ the ________ or ________ in the ________.

How is this statement supported by the lessons you have learned during this *Begin with Christ* Bible study? We have studied many aspects of this problem, so address the ones that the Holy Spirit has impressed on your heart.

John goes on to talk about "anyone [who] loves the world." What does the remainder of 1 John 2:15 say about those who love the world?

Once again, what have you learned in the *Begin with Christ* Bible study about the two kingdoms and the choices we must make daily?

First John 2:16 describes three things that do not come from the Father. The lust of the eyes is one. What are the other two?

During our Week Five study, we examined the role our eyes play with regard to temptation. How might "cravings" and "boasting" about what we have (including knowledge about diet and exercise programs!) and do be part of the things we will need to cast aside so that we can run the First Place 4 Health race set before us?

According to 1 John 2: 16, where do the things that lead us astray come from?

Loving Savior, You continue to lead me like a shepherd. Thank You for showing me the truth so that I can avoid the pitfalls that will cause me to lose sight of You. Amen.

LAVISH LOVE

Day 4

My Lord and my God, You died for me. Help me to live for You. Amen.

During Day Six of our Week Nine study, we looked at characteristics of the Kingdom of the Littles. What Littles did you circle during that exercise?

How can the knowledge of God's love for you help you overcome the things that drag you down?

According to the apostle John, there is something amazing about God's love that is in direct contrast to the Littles. Turn now to 1 John 3:1. How does John describe God's love?

What does John tell us God has done to show how lavish His love for us really is?

What does being called a child of God mean to you?

How did you become part of God's family? (Galatians 4:4-7 will help you answer this question.)

According to 1 John 3:1, why does the world not appreciate or understand the things we do to please God?

How might the beloved disciple's words be applicable to people who don't appreciate or understand why you are participating in First Place 4 Health?

Rather than trying to get other people to understand what you are doing and why you are doing it, what are you called to do? In answering this question, remember that trying to change others is one of the ways our archenemy diverts us from our appointed course. (If you are having a difficult time figuring out the answer, the last sentence of 1 John 2:27 may help you!)

The first sentence of 1 John 3:7 is a lesson we have seen repeated throughout this *Begin with Christ* Bible study:

Dear ____________, do ________ let ______________ lead you ________________.

During our Week Four study, you were asked to compile a list of those who might oppose your First Place 4 Health efforts. How can you apply the apostle John's words to give you added strength and courage in dealing with the people, places and things that threaten to lead you astray?

In our *Begin with Christ* Bible study, we have also learned about the prince of this world, our archenemy whose desire is to lead us astray. Battling against the forces of evil can be a scary proposition until we learn another important truth the apostle John is eager to teach us. Turn to 1 John 4:4. What encouragement do you get from this verse?

Because the One who is in you is stronger than the prince of this world, how have you been able to overcome the forces that continually try to drag you down?

Going back to our Week Nine study, who is the One who is in you, and what does He bring to help you in your struggle against the forces of evil?

Spend the rest of your study time today thanking God for being your source of strength and enabling you to overcome the forces of evil because Jesus has already won the battle against evil on your behalf.

O gracious and loving Lord, how fortunate I am to be a child of God. How blessed I am to have Your Holy Spirit living in me and giving me courage, love and self-discipline. Amen.

Day 5 LOVE ONE ANOTHER

O perfect Love, on my own I can do no good thing. You are the One who has shown me what it means to love. Amen.

As the short book of 1 John continues to teach us about the love of God, the beloved disciple moves his focus from loving God to loving others. Turn today to 1 John 4:7. Who does the apostle address us as?

What does John ask his dear friends to do?

Exactly where does this love we are to give others come from?

According to 1 John 4:7-8, what does our loving others demonstrate?

First John 4:9 is a confirmation of many of the truths we have studied throughout the *Begin with Christ* Bible study. Read that verse *aloud* so that you get the full impact of the apostle's words! According to 1 John 4:10, what is love?

How does this agree or disagree with what the world we live in calls love? Is God's love a romantic "in love" feeling or an everlasting commitment? Explain your answer.

Verse 11 of 1 John 4 begins, "Dear friends . . ." What is the impact of having the beloved disciple call you a dear friend?

What does John tell his dear friends in 1 John 4:11? (It is the reason we are to love one another.)

In 1 John 4:12, the beloved disciple reasons that although we have not seen God, His love lives in us and can be complete in us "if we ____________ ____________." How are the apostle John's words akin to the new command Jesus gave His disciples in this week's memory verse?

In our memory verse, Jesus tells us:

All ________ will ____________ that you are my ________________, if you ____________ one another.

How does 1 John 4:19-21 expand on Jesus' new commandment?

Throughout the *Begin with Christ* Bible study, we have talked about giving practical expression to the words that proclaim that Christ has first place in our life. Give one example of a practical way you can express your love for your First Place 4 Health brothers and sisters.

How is doing everything that Jesus tells you to do part of loving others in your First Place 4 Health group? Reflect on all you have learned during this study to properly answer this question!

O Lord God, You loved me and gave me an example of what love looks like. When I obey Your commands, I not only express my love for you but I also teach others how to love You in practical, tangible ways. Amen.

Day 6

REFLECTION AND APPLICATION

Lord, there is so much more I need to learn from You. Thank You for sending the Holy Spirit to remind me of Your teachings and guide me into all truth. Amen.

We have come to the next to last lesson in our *Begin with Christ* Bible study. Tomorrow we will be busy preparing for our victory celebration—and we have much to celebrate! We have learned more about Jesus and what it means to give tangible expression to our commitment to give Him top billing—supremacy—in our lives. At the beginning of this study, we determined to learn more about Jesus and about what it means to love and serve Him. The daily Bible studies were crafted to teach you about God's love for you and to show you how you can express your love for Him, too.

Today, during this day of reflection and application, recap what you have learned during this study, using your spiritual journal to herald your progress. Tell what you have learned about Jesus as if you were explaining it to someone who asked you about God's lavish love. Be sure to include what God, in Christ, has done for you on a practical level as you have participated in the First Place 4 Health program.

Also, be sure to write about how loving self-care is part of showing your love for God—an expression of His love for you and yours for Him. Conclude your writing by affirming again that Jesus is the Lord of your life; He is the One who died to give you eternal life. If you are not sure about your commitment to Christ, you might want to reread some of the Week Seven lessons, especially Day Four, in which you were invited to confess Christ as your Lord and Savior.

To help you realize just how much progress you have made during this First Place 4 Health session, revisit the assessment you did at the beginning of this study. As you did in that prior assessment, rate yourself on a scale from 1 to 5, with 1 being the weakest and 5 the strongest:

Physical Strength, Stamina and Stability	1	2	3	4	5
Emotional Strength, Stamina and Stability	1	2	3	4	5
Mental Strength, Stamina and Stability	1	2	3	4	5
Spiritual Strength, Stamina and Stability	1	2	3	4	5

Now turn back in your *Begin with Christ* Bible study book and see what your prior assessment looked like. What did you discover?

Thank You, Lord Christ, for loving me and giving Yourself for me so that I can be part of the wonderful family of God. Amen.

Day 7

REFLECTION AND APPLICATION

O Lord God, You deserve all the glory, honor and praise for all that I say and do because it is only by the power of Your Holy Spirit working in me that I can do any good thing. Amen.

Congratulations! Not only did you begin this journey to health and wholeness, but you have also completed a Bible study designed to teach you about Jesus, the One deserving of first place in your life! Perhaps this is the first Bible study you have managed to complete. If that is true, affirm yourself for making the commitment and taking the time to put your words into practice. Also remember to give God thanks and praise for allowing you to complete the good work you began!

Much like the ancient Israelites built altars and worshiped God each time they reached a faith milestone, it is important that you acknowledge God for His goodness and grace through this session of First Place 4 Health. During your group's victory celebration next week, you will be asked to briefly share what you have learned through this session. Today, begin to consider the highs and lows you have experienced through the last 11 weeks and how you have seen God's hand working in your First Place 4 Health journey. Write about these in the space below or in your spiritual journal.

Group Prayer Requests

first place 4 health

Today's Date: ______________________

Name	Request

Results

Week Twelve

time to celebrate!

To help you shape your brief victory celebration testimony, prayerfully work through the following questions in your spiritual journal, one on each day leading up to your group's celebration:

Day One: List some of the benefits you have gained by allowing the Lord to transform your life through this 12-week First Place 4 Health session. Be mindful that He has been active in all four aspects of your being, so list benefits you have received in the physical, mental, emotional and spiritual realms.

Day Two: In what ways have you most significantly changed mentally? Have you seen a shift in the ways you think about yourself, food, your relationships or God? How has Scripture memory been a part of these shifts?

Day Three: In what ways have you most significantly changed emotionally? Have you begun to identify how your feelings influence your relationship to food and exercise? What are you doing to stay aware of your emotions, both positive and negative?

Day Four: In what ways have you most significantly changed spiritually? How has your relationship with God deepened? How has drawing closer to Him made a difference in the other three areas of your life?

Day Five: In what ways have you most significantly changed physically? Have you met or exceeded your weight/measurement goals? How has your health improved during the past 12 weeks?

Day Six: Was there one person in your First Place 4 Health group who was particularly encouraging to you? How did their kindness make a difference in your First Place 4 Health journey?

Day Seven: Summarize the previous six questions into a one-page testimony, or "faith story," to share at your group's victory celebration. Also include the results of your self-assessment from Day Six of last week's study.

All of us at First Place 4 Health are grateful that you have shared this *Begin with Christ* Bible study with us. We hope you will continue to journey with us, your friends and fellow travelers, as we progress down the road toward health, wholeness and a lifestyle that brings glory and honor to our Creator.

Begin with Christ leader discussion guide

For in-depth information, guidance and helpful tips about leading a successful First Place 4 Health group, spend time studying the *First Place 4 Health Leader's Guide*. In it, you will find valuable answers to most of your questions, as well as personal insights from many First Place 4 Health group leaders.

For the group meetings in this session, be sure to read and consider each week's discussion topics several days before the meeting—some questions and activities require supplies and/or planning to complete. Also, if you are leading a large group, plan to break into smaller groups for discussion and then come together as a large group to share your answers and responses. Make sure to appoint a capable leader for each small group so that discussions stay focused and on track (and be sure each group records their answers!).

week one: welcome to *Begin with Christ*

During this first week, welcome the members to your group, provide a brief overview of the First Place 4 Health program, explain what is expected of the participants at each of the weekly meetings, and collect the Member Surveys. (See the *First Place 4 Health Leader's Guide* for a detailed outline of how to conduct the first week's meeting.)

week two: getting to know Him

As you and the group begin to work through the *Begin with Christ* Bible study, be mindful that there may be those in your group who have not done a focused Bible study before. Be sure to take some time at the beginning of this week's lesson time to explain the importance of daily Bible study as an integral part of First Place 4 Health.

At the beginning of the study, participants were also asked to make an assessment of where they currently are in the four facets of their being. Spend time talking about the importance of balance—and ask members who are willing to do so to share the results of their assessment.

Talk with your group about the word "supremacy" from the Day One lesson. You might want to put "supremacy" on a whiteboard or flip chart, and record what mental pictures the word brings up for people in your group.

To fully understand the wonder of grace, people must realize what Jesus has saved them from. Give your group time to share parts of their diet horror stories and how Jesus has rescued them from the deceptions and enslavements of the past.

Talk about Jesus, the great high priest, the One who intercedes for us. Ask your group what weaknesses they need to bring to the great high priest today, and then lead a time of prayer to present these needs before the throne of grace.

The "I Am" statements of Jesus will be used throughout this study. Go over the "I Am" verses and be sure your folks understand what each one means.

Lead a discussion on what doubts and fears are keeping the people in your group from declaring Jesus as the risen Savior, their Lord and their God.

Put the words "You Are" on your whiteboard or flip chart. Ask the group what responses they had to Jesus' question. Be sure that everyone has an opportunity to share at least one "You Are" statement, and record the answers.

Ask each member of your group to share one new thing he or she learned about Jesus during this week's study.

week three: pray for spiritual stamina and strength

Begin your session this week with prayer! That is the topic of our lessons, and nothing helps folks better understand prayer than praying.

Worry is something we all battle. Ask your group, "What can you change by worrying?" Have someone record the answers given on the whiteboard or flip chart. Follow your discussion by reading Matthew 6:34.

Have someone in your group read aloud 1 Peter 5:6-9. On the whiteboard or flip chart, list the four instructions we are given at the beginning of each verse, and discuss each one.

Ask your group, "Why is it essential that we allow God to bear our burdens daily?" Relate this daily unburdening to an important way our gracious God takes care of all our needs.

Micah 6:8 tells us to do three things. List those three things on your whiteboard or flip chart, and then talk about how each of those three things is a necessary ingredient in the First Place 4 Health program.

Have your group recite in unison Proverbs 3:5-8. Be sure to have extra copies of these verses so that everyone reads from the same Bible translation.

Proverbs 3:8 contains a wonderful promise for those of us who suffer from the ill effects of out-of-control eating. Ask your group what we must do before that promise becomes ours. (The answer is contained in the Proverbs 3:5-8 passage!)

Our memory verse for this week can easily be misinterpreted. Be sure to stress the importance of praying in sync with God's will and way rather than believing that our self-indulgent prayers will be fulfilled.

Ask each member of your group to share the activity they did for the prayer-in-motion exercise on Day Seven. Be sure that they talk about why they chose this movement, and how prayer in motion is different from praying while sitting in stillness.

week four: joyful obedience is the pathway to blessing

This week's lesson is about obedience, but in order to be obedient to God's commands, we must first eliminate those things that stand between us and that obedience. Spend some time talking about the following:

1. Outer things that hinder
2. Inner things that entangle

You might want to list both of these things on your whiteboard or flip chart, and brainstorm with your group about what these things are in their lives.

In order to be obedient, we must persevere. One-time obedience, followed by a season of disobedience, does not please God. Talk to your group about the importance of taking the next right step in the right direction rather than taking one step forward and two steps back.

Talk to your group about the difference between joyful obedience and grudging obedience (that is, grumbling and complaining as you obey).

Hebrews 12:2 describes Jesus as the author and perfecter of our faith. Put the words "author" and "perfecter" on your whiteboard or flip chart, then talk about how these words are different and how they are the same. The concept of the "author of the script" and the "director of the play" give a good analogy.

During the Day Four lesson, participants were asked to identify the joy set before them in the physical, mental, emotional and spiritual realms. Ask your group to share what joy in each of these areas looks like to them.

Lead a discussion about the difference between perseverance and immediate gratification.

Day Five's lesson asked your group to identify people who might oppose their First Place 4 Health efforts. Be sure to spend ample time on this subject. Unless your group members can identify the opposition they will face as they persevere, they will grow weary and lose heart.

Have your group make their own "Open During Remodeling" and "Please Watch Your Step" signs. As they do so, ask each person to share how God is remodeling their life and what it feels like to still be in the world during the process. Have fun with this exercise!

week five: our folly and God's forgiveness

This week's lessons have been about God's unconditional forgiveness. It is likely that there will be people in your class who are burdened with guilt and shame. Be sensitive to their pain.

We began our study of sin "in the beginning." Go back to the Genesis story of the fall of humanity. Read Genesis 3:1-3 and identify the four people who were in the garden that fateful day.

Ask your group to look at Eve's two mistakes. (The first was to have a conversation with Satan; the second was to alter God's words.) Be sure your group understands that when we try to argue with Satan, we set ourselves up to fail.

One of the Day Two questions asked that participants think of creative ways to keep their eyes from leading them into temptation. Ask the group what they came up with. Write the responses on the whiteboard or flip chart.

Adam and Eve hid from the Lord because they were ashamed. Ask your group how they hide when they have not been faithful to eat healthful, nutritious food.

Talk about The Genesis 3:12 Defense. Ask group members to identify a time when they blamed someone else rather than took personal responsibility for eating something not on the Live It plan.

Ask someone to read aloud 2 Chronicles 16:9, and ask another to recite the memory verse for the week. Lead a discussion about God's eyes and how the fact that the Lord's eyes roam the earth can be a source of comfort and a source of despair. Do not spend your entire meeting talking about sin. Instead, save time to talk about God's marvelous forgiveness. Being weighed down by sin can fuel compulsive eating. Read aloud the wonderful words found in 1 John 1:8-10 that give assurance of pardon.

Ask two or three people in your group to share the "right-way instant-replay" they wrote for their Day Seven assignment. Ask the group to identify the feelings that success brings.

End your session with the words of Psalm 139:23-24 as the closing prayer.

week six: God's truth and temptation's lie

Temptation is the thing that stands between most of us and success in First Place 4 Health! During this week's study we have learned some predictable-pattern truths about how Satan works. On your whiteboard or flip chart, write the words "Temptation's Lie." Brainstorm with your group the various ways our archenemy deceives us.

Temptation always follows commitment! Ask two or three people in your group to talk about how they have seen this pattern play itself out in their commitment to healthy eating.

Jesus was tempted in three different ways:

1. Provision
2. Protection
3. Power

Ask your group how these three things are ways that Satan tempts them, too. Many in First Place 4 Health come from a background where scarcity and fear were the norm. It is important for your folks to realize that Satan will use memories of past deprivation and abuse to lead them into temptation.

Talk to your group about the importance of Scripture memory as a defense against temptation and as the means God often provides for our escape. Ask your group to share a time when they were about to weaken and suddenly a Scripture verse came to mind.

On Day Five, participants were asked to remember how their First Place 4 Health group has ministered to them when they were weak or being tempted—or both. Have each member in your group affirm the others for being their God-sent angels to help in their time of need.

Don't end your session on the topic of temptation. Switch to God's faithfulness. On your whiteboard or flip chart, write "God's Faithfulness," and spend the rest of your lesson time listening to the stories of how God has indeed been faithful to members of your group.

End the session with thanksgiving and praise to the One who is always faithful. If you or someone in your group is musical, sing a praise song!

week seven: spiritual food for spiritual life

This week was a turning point in our *Begin with Christ* Bible study as participants were asked to make a commitment for Christ. If anyone in your group accepted Christ for the first time, be sure to plan a celebration time. The angels in heaven are rejoicing and we should rejoice, too!

It is important that in order to fully understand this week's memory verse, your group members comprehend the three different types of life found in the Bible, represented by the one word in our English language. On your whiteboard or flip chart, write the three types of life:

1. *Bios*
2. *Psuche*
3. *Zoe*

Lead a discussion about these three different words for "life" and what they signify. This is a vital concept, so spend ample time in discussion.

Have a member of your group read aloud the story of Nicodemus in John 3:1-18. Use this story to illustrate why we must distinguish between the physical, emotional and spiritual realms of our being.

Balance is an important part of First Place 4 Health. Lead a discussion about how the four different facets of our being are separate and how they are connected. We can't expect to do well in one area when the other parts are still out of control. Use the example of putting four different shades of food coloring in the same glass of water to illustrate how the four sides of our person are interconnected.

Talk about the connection between Jesus the living Word and Jesus the bread of life. Remind your group that when Jesus shared the Last Supper with His disciples, He broke the bread and said that it was His body, which must be broken and crucified for our sins (see Luke 22:19). In the same way, we must break open the Word to benefit from the spiritual nutrition it contains.

On Day Seven, participants were asked to go through the weeks of study thus far and list positive ways each week's lessons have impacted their First Place 4 Health participation. Next, participants were to write about how they have applied in a practical way the lessons learned. Spend time going over this chart, and ask your group to share their lessons and applications.

Be sure to be available to answer questions and hear the prayer of any in your group who are ready to accept Christ as their Lord and Savior in your meeting!

week eight: radical transformation

One of the things we need to continually combat is the quick-fix mentality of those who want instant results. Open your session by talking about the futility of diet-and-exercise programs that offer instant results. Keep in mind, though, that there may be some in your group who have resorted to gastric bypass surgery or other drastic measures. Be careful not to be condemning.

Talk with your group about the connection between not conforming to the world and being able to discern the Lord's will. Many people say they know God's will, but until they have allowed the Lord to transform their mind, knowing God's will simply is not possible.

Select four people from your group to read aloud from a different Bible translation this week's memory verse. Use the *New International Version, THE MESSAGE, The New Testament in Modern English* by J. B. Phillips, and the *New Living Translation.* (These are all in the study book.) Have your group discuss what they learned from each one of these translations that they would not have learned by just reading one Bible version.

It is easy to become too well-adjusted to our instant-results society. Ask your group to identify faulty ideas they still have about diet and exercise. Record the group's ideas on your whiteboard or flip chart.

The J. B. Phillips translation of the Bible tells us not to let the world squeeze us into its mold. Have your group members share about how they have tried to squeeze themselves into ill-fitting clothing in an attempt to be fashionable.

If you can find a small seed (ideally, a mustard seed), bring it to class. Talk about how this tiny seed will grow into a large plant. Compare it to small faith that grows over time.

The ladder exercise during the Day Five study is another invitation for your group to talk about the spiritual growth process. If members are willing to share where they are on the ladder, ask them to do so.

On Day Seven, the group members completed an exercise in which they were to describe, in some way or another, how the world drags them down and how God brings out the best of them. Ask each member in the group to share what he or she created.

week nine: filled with the Spirit

Being "filled with the Spirit" means different things to different denominations. Note that our study this week did not cover spiritual gifts but rather focused on the gift we all receive: the Holy Spirit! Try to avoid controversial aspects of the Spirit and focus on the benefits we all agree are part of the Spirit's ministry.

Begin the session by having the group recite in unison this week's memory verse. Then ask the group about the price we were bought at and who paid it!

Before the meeting, go through your own study book and list all the benefits the Spirit brings when He takes up residence in our heart. During the meeting, ask group members to identify the benefits the Spirit gives us. Write these answers on your whiteboard or flip chart. Compare answers to your list to be sure they have all been listed. Ask each group member to identify one truth the Spirit led them into this week.

Be sure to emphasize that now that Jesus is with us in Spirit (rather than a physical body), He is *always* with us—we are never abandoned or left orphans! Be sure to stop and praise God when you talk about this truth.

Before your meeting, ask someone in your group who has gone through a recent time of sadness or loss to talk to your group about how difficult it was to pray when burdened with grief. Stress that the Spirit prays for us when we can't pray for ourselves.

Proverbs 23:19-21 tells a truth that most of us would prefer to ignore. Read this proverb aloud, and then talk about all the different sins of excess—and how they are all one and the same before God. Talk about how indulgent eating leaves us drowsy and "in rags." Ask two or three members of your group to talk about the Kingdom of the Littles exercise and which two Littles they picked as still being problematic for them. Brainstorm with the group how these two Littles are interrelated. End your session by singing a hymn of praise!

week ten: more commitment

Begin this session by talking about the two kingdoms and two rulers who vie for our attention. On your whiteboard or flip chart, write "Kingdom of Darkness" and "Kingdom of Light." Lead a group discussion about the benefits of God's kingdom and the dangers found in the kingdom of the world.

Write the word "Commit" across the top of your whiteboard or flip chart. Ask group members to give some of the definitions of the word "commit" they found when they looked up the word in the dictionary.

Stress that when a commitment is made to First Place 4 Health, that commitment is actually made to two people: *God* and *self*. If we have not been faithful to that commitment, those are the two people we have failed!

God committed to do four things for the Israelites when He brought them out of Egypt. Ask the group to identify those four things and then talk about how they have application to the First Place 4 Health program.

Read Ecclesiastes 4:9-12 and then go through, item by item, the benefits of having a companion (or companions) on the journey to health and fitness.

Have someone in your group read 1 Samuel 7:3 aloud. Lead a discussion about what the people had to do before God's promise to them would become reality. Ask how that same "if-then" principle applies to our First Place 4 Health efforts.

Doing good in the face of opposition is difficult. Ask your group to talk about the people who have made their commitment to First Place 4 Health difficult, and how each participant has persevered in doing good, even in the presence of opposition.

Ask the group members if they have committed to the First Place 4 Health program for one year, and how making this commitment will be part of their First Place 4 Health success.

week eleven: love defines discipleship

Begin your session this week with a reminder that your group is deeply loved by God. Consider writing "love notes" ahead of time—note cards with Scripture verses—from God to each member.

Lead a discussion about the danger of putting God's love to the test. Ask your members to share how they have tried in the past to test God's love instead of trusting and responding to Him.

On a whiteboard or flip chart, label three columns "Past," "Present" and "Future." Ask your group to share ways that God's love for them has been, is or will be demonstrated in each time period. Have a volunteer record the answers on the board or chart.

Have someone in your group read aloud 1 John 2:15-17. Lead a discussion about how these verses relate to what your group has learned through this study. Focus on the contrast between loving the world and loving God.

Ask your group, "What does it mean to be a child of God?" List benefits and requirements of being a part of God's family on the whiteboard or flip chart.

Read 1 John 4:4 aloud. Ask your group to share some specific ways they have been able to overcome the forces of the evil one through the power of the One who lives within them.

Ask your group to read 1 John 4:9-10 aloud together three times. Between each reading, sit in silence together for 10 or 15 seconds to let the words sink into each person's heart.

Now have one person read 1 John 4:11 in response to the group's reading. Ask your members to share some practical ways they can follow this command to love each other. List these on the whiteboard or flip chart.

End the discussion with an invitation to obey the command to love each other this week. Ask your members to pick one of the activities listed to express their love for another group member before next week's victory celebration.

week twelve: time to celebrate!

Even though most of your meeting this week will be a victory celebration, take time to talk about how much God loves us and how we are called to love our brothers and sisters in Christ because God loves us. (See "Planning a Victory Celebration" in the *First Place 4 Health Leader's Guide* for ideas about throwing a successful celebration for your group.)

During the past week, each member of your group will have prepared a *Begin with Christ* faith story. Spend time giving members an equal opportunity to share the good things God has done for them in this First Place 4 Health session. Don't allow the more talkative group members to monopolize all the time. Even the quiet members need an opportunity to share their stories! Be sure members share the progress they have made, as reflected in the self-assessment done at the beginning of this Bible study and again on Day Six of Week Eleven.

End your victory celebration with the prayer found at the end of Week Eleven, Day Seven.

First Place 4 Health menu plans

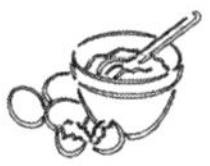

Each menu plan is based on approximately 1,400 to 1,500 calories per day. All recipe and menu exchanges were determined using the MasterCook software, a program that accesses a database containing more than 6,000 food items prepared using the United States Department of Agriculture (USDA) publications and information from food manufacturers. As with any nutritional program, MasterCook calculates the nutritional values of the recipes based on ingredients. Nutrition may vary due to how the food is prepared, where the food comes from, soil content, season, ripeness, processing and method of preparation. For these reasons, please use the recipes and menu plans as approximate guides. As always, consult your physician and/or a registered dietitian before starting a weight-loss program.

For those who need more calories, add the following to the 1,400-calorie plan:

- 1,800 calories: 2 ounce equivalent of meat, 3 ounce equivalent of bread, 1/2 cup vegetable serving, 1 tsp. fat
- 2,000 calories: 2 ounce equivalent of meat, 4 ounce equivalent of bread, 1/2 cup vegetable serving, 3 tsp. fat
- 2,200 calories: 2 ounce equivalent of meat, 5 ounce equivalent of bread, 1/2 cup vegetable serving, 1/2 cup fruit serving, 5 tsp. fat
- 2,400 calories: 2 ounce equivalent of meat, 6 ounce equivalent of bread, 1 cup vegetable serving, 1/2 cup fruit serving, 6 tsp. fat

First Week Grocery List

Produce

- ❑ (1) bag green grapes
- ❑ (1) bag celery stalks
- ❑ (1) apple
- ❑ (2) plums
- ❑ (1) orange
- ❑ (1) peach
- ❑ (5) potatoes
- ❑ (1) banana
- ❑ 3/4 cup blueberries
- ❑ (1) honeydew melon
- ❑ 1 cup raspberries
- ❑ (1) small mango
- ❑ 1 cup strawberries
- ❑ 4 cups snap beans
- ❑ (2) bunches broccoli
- ❑ (1) bunch cilantro
- ❑ 2 1/8 tbsp. lime juice
- ❑ (4) jalapeno peppers
- ❑ (4) red onions
- ❑ (1) bunch spinach
- ❑ 2 cups green beans
- ❑ (4) Roma tomatoes
- ❑ (1) large tomato
- ❑ 1 cup mushrooms
- ❑ (11) garlic cloves
- ❑ (10) cherry tomatoes
- ❑ (1) bunch green onions
- ❑ (1) bunch dark green lettuce
- ❑ (1) cucumber
- ❑ (1) cantaloupe
- ❑ (1) bag carrots
- ❑ (1) bag carrot sticks
- ❑ 1/4 cup fresh lemon juice

Breads and Cereals

- ❑ whole-wheat bread
- ❑ bagels
- ❑ whole-wheat English muffins
- ❑ (5) dinner rolls
- ❑ (6) breadsticks
- ❑ (1) pita bread
- ❑ (14) 6-inch low-fat tortillas
- ❑ (2) 16-ounce cans navy beans
- ❑ cornflakes
- ❑ fortified cereal of your choice
- ❑ wheat flake cereal
- ❑ saltine crackers
- ❑ brown rice

Canned Goods

- ❑ (1) 16-oz. can baked beans
- ❑ (1) 8-oz. can white meat chicken
- ❑ Healthy Choice® cream of chicken soup
- ❑ (2) 16-oz. cans low-sodium broth
- ❑ (1) can gazpacho soup
- ❑ (3) 4-oz. cans green chilies

Baking Products

- ❑ granulated sugar
- ❑ cooking wine
- ❑ coking sherry
- ❑ flour
- ❑ marjoram
- ❑ Old Bay® seafood seasoning
- ❑ cinnamon
- ❑ dried thyme
- ❑ dried onions
- ❑ paprika
- ❑ dried parsley

- ❑ lemon pepper seasoning
- ❑ cayenne pepper
- ❑ bay leaves
- ❑ Creole seasoning
- ❑ salt
- ❑ pepper
- ❑ dried oregano
- ❑ ground cumin
- ❑ Dijon mustard
- ❑ Worcestershire sauce
- ❑ vegetable oil or canola oil
- ❑ olive oil
- ❑ low-fat mayonnaise
- ❑ chunky-style spaghetti sauce
- ❑ BBQ sauce
- ❑ reduced-calorie maple-flavored syrup
- ❑ orange marmalade
- ❑ 1/4 cup salsa
- ❑ low-sodium soy sauce

Dairy Products

- ❑ 4 oz. reduced-fat Colby-Jack cheese
- ❑ 20 oz. low-fat cheddar cheese
- ❑ 2 oz. low-fat mozzarella cheese
- ❑ nonfat milk
- ❑ light margarine
- ❑ 32 oz. nonfat plain yogurt
- ❑ 10 oz. light sour cream

Seafood and Meat

- ❑ 1 1/2 lbs. cod
- ❑ 1/4 lb. shrimp
- ❑ 1/2 lb. catfish
- ❑ 1 oz. turkey bacon
- ❑ 1 oz. turkey pepperoni
- ❑ (1) reduced-fat hot dog
- ❑ low-fat Italian turkey sausage
- ❑ 2 1/2 lbs. skinless, boneless chicken breasts

Frozen Foods

- ❑ frozen whole-wheat waffles
- ❑ 2 1/2 cups frozen corn kernels
- ❑ 1/2 cup frozen broccoli flowerets

First Week Meals and Recipes

DAY 1

Breakfast

2 whole-wheat frozen waffles
1 tsp. light margarine
1 cup nonfat milk
2 tsp. reduced-calorie maple syrup
1 cup honeydew melon

Nutritional Information: 502 calories; (12% calories from fat); 2g fat; 9g protein; 32g carbohydrate; 1g dietary fiber; 4mg cholesterol; 208mg sodium; 313mg calcium.

Lunch

Veggie Cheese Quesadillas

nonstick cooking spray
2 oz. reduced-fat Colby-Jack cheese, grated
1/4 cup mushrooms, sliced
2 (6-inch) nonfat tortillas
1 tbsp. reduced-fat sour cream
1/2 cup frozen broccoli florets, cooked
1/4 cup salsa

Coat a nonstick skillet with cooking spray and heat. Put one tortilla in pan and sprinkle with cheese. Place broccoli and mushrooms on top of cheese. Cover with the second tortilla and brown on both sides. Remove from pan and let sit a minute. Slice and serve with sour cream and salsa. Serve with 1 cup carrot sticks and 1/2 cup sliced peaches in own juice.

Nutritional Information: 458 calories (13% calories from fat); 7g fat; 26g protein; 79g carbohydrate; 24g dietary fiber; 15mg cholesterol; 1,077mg sodium; 425mg calcium; 4mg iron.

Dinner

Grilled Chicken Breasts with Corn Salsa

Salsa

1 1/2 cups frozen corn kernels, thawed
1/4 cup red bell pepper, chopped
1 1/2 tbsp. fresh lime juice
1/4 cup red onion, chopped
1/4 cup fresh cilantro, chopped

Combine all ingredients in bowl. Season with salt and pepper. May be made the day before; cover and refrigerate.

Chicken

1/2 cup cooking sherry
1 tbsp. fresh cilantro, chopped
1 to 2 tsp. (to taste) jalapenos, chopped and seeded
1 tbsp. low-sodium soy sauce
2 tsp fresh lime juice
4 skinless, boneless chicken breast halves

Combine first five ingredients in medium bowl. Add chicken and turn to coat. Cover and refrigerate at least 1 hour or up to 4 hours. Preheat barbecue (medium-high heat) or broiler. Drain chicken, season with salt and pepper to taste. Grill or broil chicken until cooked through, about 4 minutes per side. Cut chicken into thin diagonal slices. Arrange chicken on plates. Top with salsa and serve. Serve with spinach salad with sliced mushrooms and tomatoes, 1 cup cooked green beans mixed with a little salsa and a dinner roll with 1 tsp. reduced-calorie margarine per person.

Nutritional Information: 412 calories (10% calories from fat); 4g fat; 59g protein; 27g carbohydrate; 4g dietary fiber; 137mg cholesterol; 362mg sodium; 74mg calcium; 4mg iron.

DAY 2

Breakfast

1 small (2 oz.) whole-wheat English muffin, split and toasted
1 cup nonfat milk
1 tsp. light margarine
1 cup strawberries, sliced

Nutritional Information: 290 calories (13% calories from fat); 4g fat; 15g protein; 50g carbohydrate; 8g dietary fiber; 4mg cholesterol; 594mg sodium; 501mg calcium; 2 mg iron.

Lunch

Soup and Salad

1 serving of canned gazpacho
2 plums
2 (1-oz.) breadsticks, topped with 2 oz. reduced-fat Colby-Jack cheese, shredded

Nutritional Information: 451 calories (21% calories from fat); 10g fat; 29g protein; 61g carbohydrate; 2g dietary fiber; 12mg cholesterol; 1,459mg sodium; 277 calcium; 2mg iron.

Dinner

Spicy White Bean and Chicken Chili

2 cans (16-oz.) navy beans
1 extra-large onion, chopped
1/2 tsp. dried oregano, crumbled
3/4 lb. boneless, skinless chicken breast, well-trimmed, cut in large pieces
3/4 cup plain nonfat yogurt
3 jalapenos, minced (optional)
2 cans (4-oz.) green chilies, diced
2 tsp. olive oil
8 large garlic cloves, minced
5 1/4 cups canned unsalted chicken broth
fresh cilantro, chopped
1 tbsp. ground cumin
3/4 cup water

Heat oil in large, heavy pot over medium heat. Add onion and garlic and sauté until tender, about 10 minutes. Stir in cumin and oregano and cook 1 minute. Mix in beans and chilies, then chicken, broth and water. Simmer until beans are very tender and chili is creamy, about 1 hour and 45 minutes or less. (*Note:* May be made 3 days ahead. Cover and refrigerate. Reheat when ready to serve.) Ladle chili into bowls. Garnish with yogurt, cilantro and minced chilies and serve immediately. Serve with a spinach salad with reduced-calorie dressing. Serves 4.

Nutritional Information: 549 calories (23% calories from fat); 16g fat; 57g protein; 62g carbohydrate; 13g dietary fiber; 1mg cholesterol; 1,109mg sodium; 287mg calcium; 9mg iron.

DAY 3

Breakfast

1 cup fortified cold cereal
1 cup nonfat milk
1/2 small mango

Nutritional Information: 263 calories (6% calories from fat); 2g fat; 12g protein; 53g carbohydrate; 5g dietary fiber; 4mg cholesterol; 348mg sodium; 313mg calcium.

Lunch

Chicken Patty Melt

2 slices whole-wheat bread
2 tsp. reduced-fat mayonnaise
1 oz. canned white chicken meat
1 oz. shredded part-skim mozzarella cheese

Toast bread. Combine chicken, mayonnaise and cheese in small bowl, and spread on toasted bread. Broil open-faced until bubbly. Serve with 1 cup of celery sticks, 1 tbsp. fat-free Ranch dressing and 1 medium apple.

Nutritional Information: 477 calories (25% calories from fat); 14g fat; 23g protein; 69g carbohydrate; 12g dietary fiber; 36mg cholesterol; 1,041mg sodium; 331mg calcium; 4mg iron.

Dinner

Lite Chicken Enchiladas

1 (8 oz.) container light sour cream
1 (10 1/2 oz.) can Healthy Choice cream of chicken soup
1 1/2 cups cooked chicken, chopped
1 cup reduced-fat cheddar cheese, shredded
nonstick cooking spray
1 (4 oz.) can green chilies, diced
12 (6-inch) low-fat tortillas
1 (8 oz.) container plain nonfat yogurt
1/4 cup green onions, sliced

Heat oven to 350° F. Spray a 13x9-inch (3-quart) baking dish with cooking spray. In medium bowl, combine sour cream, yogurt, soup and chilies, mix well. Spoon about 3 tbsp. sour cream mixture down the center of each tortilla. Reserve $1/4$ cup of cheddar cheese; sprinkle each tortilla with remaining cheese, chicken and onions. Roll tortillas and place in spray-coated dish, seam side down. Spoon remaining sour-cream mixture over tortillas. Cover with foil and bake 25 to 30 minutes, or until hot and bubbly. Remove foil, sprinkle with reserved $1/4$ cup cheese. Return to oven uncovered and bake an additional 5 minutes or until cheese is melted. Serve enchiladas on top of shredded lettuce and chopped tomatoes with $1/2$ cup salsa per person. Serves 6.

Nutritional Information: 743 calories (23% calories from fat); 19g fat; 49g protein; 95g carbohydrate; 7g dietary fiber; 68mg cholesterol; 2,173mg sodium; 477mg calcium; 5mg iron.

DAY 4

Breakfast

1 slice whole-wheat bread, toasted and topped with 1 tsp. light margarine and $1/2$ tsp. granulated sugar and pinch of cinnamon
$3/4$ cup nonfat plain vanilla yogurt mixed with $3/4$ cup blueberries

Nutritional Information: 319 calories (13% calories from fat); 5g fat; 16g protein; 56g carbohydrate; 7g dietary fiber; 3mg cholesterol; 478mg sodium; 388mg calcium; 2mg iron.

Lunch

Veggie Pizza

1 (6-inch) flat pita bread
$1/4$ cup broccoli florets
$1/4$ cup prepared chunky-style spaghetti sauce
1 oz. part-skim mozzarella, shredded
$1/4$ cup carrots, shredded
$1/4$ cup tomatoes, diced
8 turkey pepperoni slices

Preheat oven to 450° F. Place pita bread on a cookie sheet. Spread sauce on top of bread. Layer with remaining ingredients, finishing with the cheese. Bake 8 to 10 minutes or until cheese is melted and bubbly. Serve with 1 small orange.

Nutritional Information: 477 calories (24% calories from fat); 13g fat; 25g protein; 66g carbohydrate; 9g dietary fiber; 53mg cholesterol; 1,368mg sodium; 348mg calcium; 3mg iron.

Dinner

Quick Baked Fish

$1\frac{1}{2}$ lbs. cod, tilapia, catfish or haddock fillets
2 tsp. dried onion flakes
1 tsp. Old Bay seasoning
$1/4$ cup low-fat mayonnaise
1 tsp. Dijon mustard
1 tsp. white wine Worcestershire sauce
$1/4$ tsp. paprika

1 tbsp. dried (or 2 tbsp. fresh, chopped) parsley
1/8 tsp. cayenne pepper
1/2 tsp. lemon pepper
nonstick cooking spray

Preheat oven to 400° F. Spray a shallow casserole dish with cooking spray; set aside. Wash fillets with cold water and pat dry with paper towels. Place fish fillets in prepared dish. In a small bowl, combine remaining ingredients until well mixed. Spread mixture evenly over fillets. Bake uncovered for 15 minutes or until fish flakes easily with a fork. Serve with steamed broccoli and 1/2 cup cooked brown rice and one breadstick per person. Serves 4.

Nutritional Information: 431 calories (21% calories from fat); 12g fat; 39g protein; 58g carbohydrate; 7g dietary fiber; 104mg cholesterol; 644mg sodium; 116mg calcium; 3mg iron.

DAY 5

Breakfast

3/4 cup corn flakes
1 cup nonfat milk
1/2 medium banana, sliced

Nutritional Information: 293 calories (3% calories from fat); 1g fat; 12g protein; 62g carbohydrate; 3g dietary fiber; 4mg cholesterol; 574mg sodium; 308mg calcium; 13mg iron.

Lunch

BBQ Franks and Beans

1 reduced-fat, all-beef frank, diced
1 tbsp. prepared BBQ sauce
1 cup baked beans, drained

Combine all ingredients. Microwave for 2 to 3 minutes. Serve with 1 cup cantaloupe cubes, and 1 cup peeled and sliced cucumber tossed with 1 tbsp. light Italian dressing.

Nutritional Information: 430 calories (6% calories from fat); 3g fat; 19g protein; 95g carbohydrate; 18g dietary fiber; 0mg cholesterol; 1,349mg sodium; 198 mg calcium; 3mg iron.

Dinner

Marmalade Chicken

1/4 cup orange marmalade
1/4 cup white cooking wine
1/4 tsp. dried thyme, crumbled
1/4 cup fresh lemon juice
1 tbsp. soy sauce, diluted with 1 tbsp. water
1 (3-lb.) chicken, cut into 4 pieces

Combine first 5 ingredients in large bowl. Remove any visible fat from chicken, but leave skin on. Add chicken to bowl with marinade; toss to coat. Cover and refrigerate 4 hours or overnight, stirring occasionally. Preheat oven to 400° F.

Place a wire rack on top of a baking sheet. Remove chicken from marinade, reserving marinade. Place chicken skin-side up on rack. Bake 20 minutes. Turn and bake 20 minutes longer. Turn chicken skin-side up and continue cooking until skin is golden brown and chicken is almost cooked through, approximately 10 minutes. Meanwhile, boil marinade in small, heavy saucepan until reduced to glaze, about 10 minutes. Remove skin and brush chicken with glaze. Bake chicken until glaze is set and chicken is cooked through, approximately 5 minutes. Serve with 1 cup roasted potatoes, 1 cup sautéed snap peas and 1 dinner roll per person. Serves 4.

Nutritional Information: 573 calories (6% calories from fat); 4g fat; 38g protein; 96g carbohydrate; 11g dietary fiber; 69mg cholesterol; 525mg sodium; 143mg calcium; 7mg iron.

DAY 6

Breakfast

1 small (2 oz.) bagel, toasted and topped with 1 tsp. light margarine
3/4 cup raspberries
1 cup nonfat milk

Nutritional Information: 287 calories (11% calories from fat); 4g fat; 14g protein; 50g carbohydrate; 10g dietary fiber; 4mg cholesterol; 410mg sodium; 364mg calcium; 2mg iron.

Lunch

Stuffed Potato

1 (6-oz.) potato, baked
1/4 cup tomato, diced
1 tsp. light margarine
1/4 cup cooked broccoli florets
1 tbsp. fat-free sour cream
1 oz. turkey bacon, cooked and crumbled
1 tbsp. green onions, diced
1 oz. reduced-fat cheddar cheese, shredded
1/4 cup mushrooms, sliced

Slice open the baked potato and scoop out insides into a small bowl. Combine with remaining ingredients and mix well. Fill shell with the mixture. Microwave until hot. Serve with 15 grapes.

Nutritional Information: 392 calories (22% calories from fat); 10g fat; 19g protein; 61g carbohydrate; 7g dietary fiber; 33mg cholesterol; 628mg sodium; 214mg calcium; 2mg iron.

Dinner

Argentine Corn Chicken

1 lb. boneless chicken breasts, skinless, cut into chunks
1/4 tsp. leaf marjoram
2 cloves garlic, minced
pepper, freshly ground, to taste
1/2 medium onion, chopped

1 tbsp. canola oil
10 whole cherry tomatoes
1 bay leaf
1 large tomato, seeded, chopped
1 cup frozen whole-kernel corn, thawed
salt

Season chicken lightly with salt and pepper. In a large nonstick skillet, heat oil. Add chicken and cook until tender, turning occasionally to prevent burning. Remove from skillet and set aside; keep warm. Sauté onion and garlic in skillet. Add chopped tomato, bay leaf and marjoram; simmer 10 minutes. Add corn, whole cherry tomatoes and chicken to skillet and heat through, mixing well. Serve each with $^{1}/_{3}$ cup brown rice and 1 cup steamed vegetables. Serves 4.

Nutritional Information: 426 calories (35% calories from fat); 17g fat; 36g protein; 37g carbohydrate; 8g dietary fiber; 0mg cholesterol; 50mg sodium.

DAY 7

Breakfast

1 cup fortified cold cereal
1 cup nonfat milk
$^{1}/_{2}$ medium banana, sliced

Nutritional Information: 254 calories (9% calories from fat); 2g fat 12g protein; 49g carbohydrate; 4g dietary fiber; 4mg cholesterol; 411mg sodium; calcium 361mg; 8mg iron.

Lunch

McDonald's® Happy Meal™
Diet soda
Tossed green salad with fat-free salad dressing

Nutritional Information: 524 calories (38% calories from fat); 22g fat; 18g protein; 65g carbohydrate; 8g dietary fiber; 25mg cholesterol; 673mg sodium; 169mg calcium; 2mg iron.

Dinner

Seafood and Turkey Sausage Gumbo

$^{1}/_{4}$ cup all-purpose flour
3 garlic cloves, chopped
1 cup canned low-salt chicken or vegetable broth
$^{1}/_{4}$ pound small shrimp, de-veined
1 cup green bell pepper, chopped
10-oz. low-fat Italian turkey sausages, casings removed
1 cup chopped onion
1 bay leaf
1 can (28-oz.) tomatoes in juice, diced
1 tbsp. vegetable oil
1 tsp. dried thyme
2 tsp. Creole or Cajun seasoning
2 (4-oz.) catfish fillets, each cut into 4 pieces

Sprinkle flour over bottom of heavy, large pot. Stir flour constantly over medium-low heat until flour turns golden brown (do not allow to burn), about 12 to 15 minutes. Pour browned flour into bowl, set aside. Heat oil in same pot over medium heat. Add onion and bell pepper; stir 1 minute. Add sausages and sauté until brown, breaking up with back of spoon, about 5 minutes. Add browned flour. Add tomatoes with juice, broth and Creole seasoning. Bring to boil. Reduce heat, cover and simmer 20 minutes to blend flavors, stirring frequently. Add shrimp and catfish to pot and simmer until seafood is opaque in center, about 5 minutes. Discard bay leaf. Season with salt and pepper and serve. Serve over $^1/_2$ cup steamed brown rice and with a green salad mixed with 2 tbsp. reduced fat dressing and 4 saltine crackers for each person. Serves 4.

Nutritional Information: 589 calories; 23g fat (33.9% calories from fat); 37g protein; 62g carbohydrate; 7g dietary fiber; 132mg cholesterol; 1,091mg Sodium; 172mg calcium; 6 mg iron.

Second Week Grocery List

Produce

- ❑ (1) peach
- ❑ 3/4 cup blueberries
- ❑ 3/4 cup blackberries
- ❑ 2 cups strawberries
- ❑ (1) grapefruit
- ❑ (1) onion
- ❑ (9) garlic cloves
- ❑ (1) green pepper
- ❑ (1) bag carrots
- ❑ (1) package fresh parsley
- ❑ 3 lbs. snap peas
- ❑ (2) bags green grapes
- ❑ (1) bunch cilantro
- ❑ 1 tbsp. fresh lime juice
- ❑ (1) jalapeno
- ❑ (1) head cabbage
- ❑ 1 lb. mushrooms
- ❑ (1) bunch green onions
- ❑ (1) bunch green cabbage leaves
- ❑ fresh basil
- ❑ fresh ginger
- ❑ fresh rosemary
- ❑ fresh sage
- ❑ (1) red bell pepper
- ❑ (2) red onions
- ❑ (1) zucchini
- ❑ (1) small eggplant
- ❑ 2 tsp. fresh lemon juice
- ❑ (1) bunch broccoli
- ❑ (4) potatoes
- ❑ (1) bunch celery
- ❑ (1) large cucumber
- ❑ (1) bag baby carrots
- ❑ (1) package alfalfa sprouts
- ❑ (1) bag mixed salad greens
- ❑ (1) bunch cauliflower
- ❑ (2) apples
- ❑ (1) bunch spinach
- ❑ (2) tomatoes

Baking Products

- ❑ cooking spray
- ❑ brown sugar
- ❑ cooking wine
- ❑ Worcestershire sauce
- ❑ Dijon mustard
- ❑ mustard
- ❑ canola oil
- ❑ olive oil
- ❑ sesame oil
- ❑ sesame seeds
- ❑ low-sodium soy sauce
- ❑ teriyaki sauce
- ❑ sugar substitute
- ❑ salt
- ❑ pepper
- ❑ ground cumin
- ❑ coarse salt
- ❑ (3) cloves
- ❑ lemon pepper seasoning
- ❑ rice wine vinegar
- ❑ balsamic vinegar
- ❑ brown rice
- ❑ raisins
- ❑ strawberry jam
- ❑ all-purpose flour
- ❑ Chinese noodles
- ❑ reduced-fat mayonnaise
- ❑ low-calorie Thousand Island dressing

- ❑ reduced-fat salad dressing
- ❑ low-calorie maple syrup

Breads and Cereals

- ❑ whole-wheat bread
- ❑ English muffins
- ❑ small bagels
- ❑ sourdough bread
- ❑ whole-wheat pita bread
- ❑ French bread
- ❑ rye bread
- ❑ wheat flakes cereal
- ❑ bran flakes
- ❑ raisin bran
- ❑ (6) low-fat 7-inch flour tortillas
- ❑ saltine crackers

Canned Foods

- ❑ (1) can fruit cocktail in juice
- ❑ (1) can pineapple chunks
- ❑ (1) can tuna in water
- ❑ (1) can tomatoes
- ❑ (1) can sauerkraut
- ❑ (1) can mixed vegetables
- ❑ (1) can Mandarin oranges
- ❑ (2) cans chicken broth
- ❑ (1) can beef broth

Dairy Products

- ❑ reduced-fat cheddar cheese
- ❑ 6 oz. reduced-fat Swiss cheese
- ❑ reduced-fat Monterey-Jack cheese
- ❑ nonfat milk
- ❑ light margarine
- ❑ 20 oz. nonfat plain yogurt
- ❑ light sour cream

Seafood and Meat

- ❑ 1 lb. large fresh uncooked shrimp
- ❑ 2 oz. sliced lean roast beef
- ❑ 2 lbs. sirloin steaks, trimmed
- ❑ 12 oz. 98% fat-free smoked turkey
- ❑ $1^1/_4$ lbs. boneless skinless chicken breasts
- ❑ 4 skinless chicken breasts (bone-in)
- ❑ $1^1/_2$ oz. corned beef
- ❑ 2 oz. cooked turkey breast

Frozen Foods

- ❑ (1) 11-oz. lean frozen dinner entrée
- ❑ Lean Cuisine® Pasta Alfredo
- ❑ frozen pancakes
- ❑ 4 cups Oriental vegetables

Second Week Meals and Recipes

DAY 1

Breakfast

2 slices sourdough bread, toasted and topped with1 tsp. light margarine
3/4 cup blueberries
1 cup nonfat milk

Nutritional Information: 304 calories (12% calories from fat); 4g fat; 13g protein; 53g carbohydrate; 4g dietary fiber; 4mg cholesterol; 483mg sodium; 347mg calcium; 2mg iron.

Lunch

Chef's Salad

1 cup dark, mixed salad greens
1 cup vegetables (broccoli, carrots, zucchini, onion, cauliflower, bell pepper), chopped
1 oz. reduced-fat Swiss cheese, diced
1 oz. cooked turkey, diced
3/4 cup Mandarin oranges
1 tbsp. reduced-fat dressing
8 saltines

Combine first five ingredients and toss in reduced-fat dressing.

Nutritional Information: 410 calories; 10g fat (23.1% calories from fat); 24g protein; 55g carbohydrate; 14g dietary fiber; 31mg cholesterol; 1,164mg sodium; 438mg calcium; 4mg iron.

Dinner

Smoked Turkey Quesadillas

nonstick cooking spray
12 oz. 98% fat-free smoked turkey, sliced
6 (7-inch) low-fat tortillas
fresh cilantro sprigs, stemmed
coarse salt
6 oz. low-fat Monterey-Jack cheese, grated
1/2 tsp. ground cumin
36 green grapes, halved lengthwise
1 tbsp. fresh lime juice

Place tortillas on work surface. Arrange cheese, turkey, grapes and cilantro over half of each tortilla. Sprinkle with cumin. Fold tortillas over filling. Preheat oven to 200° F. Heat large, nonstick skillet over medium heat. Coat with vegetable spray. Cook quesadillas, one at a time, until golden brown, about 3 minutes, turning once. Turn again. Brush cooked top with lime juice and sprinkle with coarse salt. Cook until golden brown, about 3 minutes. Keep warm in oven. Repeat with remaining quesadillas. Serve each with 1/4 cup chunky salsa mixed with 1 tsp. reduced-fat sour cream. Serves 6.

Nutritional Information: 483 calories (25% calories from fat); 13g fat; 24g protein; 63g carbohydrate; 5g dietary fiber; 20mg cholesterol; 888mg sodium; 650mg calcium.

DAY 2

Breakfast

1 small (2 oz.) bagel, toasted and topped with 1 tsp. strawberry jam
3/4 cup artificially sweetened mixed-berry nonfat yogurt, mixed with 3/4 cup blackberries

Nutritional Information: 310 calories (5% calories from fat); 2g fat; 16g protein; 59g carbohydrate; 7g dietary fiber; 3mg cholesterol; 409mg sodium; 413mg calcium; 3mg iron.

Lunch

Sandwich and Salad

2 slices whole-grain bread
2 oz. cooked turkey breast, sliced
1 tsp. reduced-fat mayonnaise
mustard and pickle (optional)

Serve with tossed green salad mixed with sliced tomatoes, cucumbers, carrots and peppers, 2 tbsp. fat-free salad dressing and 1/3 cup pineapple tidbits.

Nutritional Information: 374 calories (13% calories from fat); 6g fat; 25g protein; 61g carbohydrate; 10g dietary fiber; 39mg cholesterol; 554mg sodium; 156mg calcium; 6mg iron.

Dinner

Rosemary-Sage Steak

1 lb. boneless top sirloin steak, all visible fat removed

Marinade

1/2 cup onion, chopped
1 tsp. olive oil
2 tbsp. fresh (or 2 tsp. dried, crushed) rosemary, finely chopped
2 tbsp. fresh (or 2 tsp. dried, crushed) sage, finely chopped
3 medium cloves garlic, minced (or 1 1/2 tsp. bottled, minced)
3 tbsp. dry white cooking wine
1/4 tsp. salt
1/4 cup fresh lemon juice
1 tbsp. Dijon mustard
1/2 tsp. pepper

Put steak in an airtight plastic bag. In a small bowl, combine marinade ingredients. Pour into bag over steak and turn to coat evenly. Seal and refrigerate from 1 to 24 hours, turning occasionally. Preheat grill on medium-high heat. Drain steak; grill for 8 to 12 minutes per side, or until done to taste. Serve with

1 cup grilled vegetables, and a 6-ounce potato topped with 1 tsp. reduced-calorie margarine and 1 tsp. reduced-fat sour cream per person. Serves 4.

Nutritional Information: 418 calories (21% calories from fat); 10g fat; 33g protein; 52g carbohydrate; 11g dietary fiber; 67mg cholesterol; 362mg sodium; 161mg calcium; 6mg iron.

DAY 3

Breakfast

1 small (2 oz.) English muffin, toasted and topped with 1 tsp. light margarine
$^1/_2$ medium grapefruit
1 cup nonfat milk

Nutritional Information: 278 calories (11% calories from fat); 3g fat; 13g protein; 48g carbohydrate; 3g dietary fiber; 4mg cholesterol; 435mg sodium; 416mg calcium; 2mg iron.

Lunch

11 oz. lean frozen dinner entrée
1 cup fresh baby carrots
1 small apple

Nutritional Information: 424 calories (16% calories from fat); 8g fat; 20g protein; 70g carbohydrate; 9g dietary fiber; 30mg cholesterol; 711mg sodium; 273mg calcium; 1mg iron.

Dinner

Grilled Sesame Chicken

2 tbsp. sesame seeds
$^1/_4$ tsp. black pepper, freshly ground
2 tbsp. soy sauce, diluted with $1^1/_2$ tbsp. water
3 cloves garlic, crushed
1 tbsp. brown sugar
4 (3-oz.) uncooked skinless chicken breasts

Combine first five ingredients in a shallow dish. Mix well. Add chicken, turning to coat. Cover and refrigerate for at least 2 hours. Remove chicken from marinade. Grill 4 to 5 inches from medium-hot coals for 15 minutes. Turn and grill until done. Serve with 1 cup cooked noodles tossed with 1 tsp. teriyaki sauce and 1 cup sautéed Oriental vegetables per person.

Nutritional Information: 419 calories (11% calories from fat); 5g fat; 40g protein; 53g carbohydrate; 7g dietary fiber; 68mg cholesterol; 865mg sodium; 148mg calcium; 6mg iron.

DAY 4

Breakfast

1 cup wheat flakes cereal
1 cup nonfat milk
1 medium peach, sliced

Nutritional Information: 242 calories (6% calories from fat); 2g fat; 12g protein; 47g carbohydrate; 5g dietary fiber; 4mg cholesterol; 346mg sodium; 307mg calcium.

Lunch

French-Dip Roast Beef Sandwich

1 (4 oz.) loaf French bread
2 oz. lean, boneless roast beef, cooked and thinly sliced
1 cup hot, low-sodium beef broth

Cut bread loaf in half horizontally, and then cut pieces in half vertically to make 4 pieces. Place 2 of the pieces, cut side up, on each of 2 plates. Top each bread piece with 1 oz. roast beef and 1/4 cup broth. Cover each plate with plastic wrap; microwave for 30 to 45 seconds until heated through. Serve with 1 cup broccoli florets with 2 tbsp. reduced-fat Ranch dressing and 1 cup strawberries per person. Serves 2.

Nutritional Information: 388 calories (16% calories from fat); 6g fat; 21g protein; 45g carbohydrate; 10g dietary fiber; 31mg cholesterol; 667mg sodium; 133mg calcium; 3mg iron.

Dinner

Shrimp Scampi

1 lb. large fresh uncooked shrimp, de-veined
1 clove garlic, minced
1/4 tsp. black pepper, freshly ground
1/4 cup white cooking wine
1 tsp. olive oil
1 tsp. margarine, melted
1 tbsp. fresh parsley, chopped

Combine margarine, oil, garlic, cooking wine and pepper in a large bowl. Add shrimp and toss lightly to coat. Spread a single layer of shrimp in a shallow, ovensafe casserole dish. Broil shrimp approximately 4 inches from heat for 3 to 4 minutes. Turn shrimp and broil for an additional 3 to 4 minutes or until lightly browned. Sprinkle with fresh chopped parsley and serve. Serve with Lean Cuisine Pasta Alfredo and snap peas. Serves 4.

Nutritional Information: 504 calories; 12g fat (38.4% calories from fat); 31g protein; 12g carbohydrate; 6g dietary fiber; 215mg cholesterol; 235mg sodium; 336mg calcium; 2mg iron.

DAY 5

Breakfast

$3/4$ cup bran flakes cereal
1 cup nonfat milk
2 tbsp. raisins

Nutritional Information: 277 calories (5% calories from fat); 2g fat; 13g protein; 56g carbohydrate; 4g dietary fiber; 4mg cholesterol; 403mg sodium; 311mg calcium.

Lunch

Tuna Salad Pita

4 oz. water-packed tuna, drained
$1/4$ cup celery, chopped
$1/4$ tsp. lemon pepper seasoning
$1/4$ cup onion, chopped
2 tbsp. reduced-calorie mayonnaise
1 (2-oz.) whole-wheat pita
$1/2$ cup alfalfa sprouts

In small bowl, combine first five ingredients. Cut one large whole-wheat pita in half crosswise and open to form two pockets. Fill each pocket with half the tuna salad and top each portion with $1/4$ cup alfalfa sprouts. Serve with 1 cup cucumber rounds, 1 cup carrot sticks and 15 grapes.

Nutritional Information: 388 calories (16% calories from fat); 6g fat; 22g protein; 51g carbohydrate; 9g dietary fiber; 22mg cholesterol; 516mg sodium; 84mg calcium; 3mg iron.

Dinner

Green Pepper Steak

1 lb. lean sirloin steak, cut into $1/4$-inch strips
$1/4$ tsp. pepper, freshly ground
1 medium onion, sliced
1 tbsp. canola oil
1 clove garlic, finely chopped
1 large green pepper, cut in strips
2 tbsp. all-purpose flour
1 can beef broth
$1/2$ tsp. salt
1 cup canned tomatoes with juice
$1\,1/2$ tsp. Worcestershire sauce

Coat strips of round steak with flour mixed with salt and pepper. Heat oil in a large frying pan. Brown meat on all sides; drain off any fat. Add broth, tomato juice (reserving tomato pieces), onion and garlic to meat. Cover and simmer about 30 to 40 minutes or until meat is tender. Add tomato pieces, green pepper strips and Worcestershire sauce. Stir and cook 10 minutes longer. Serve over $1/2$ cup cooked brown rice and with $1/2$ cup cooked carrots per person. Serves 4.

Nutritional Information: 476 calories (37% calories from fat); 20g fat; 29g protein; 45g carbohydrate; 5g dietary fiber; 71mg cholesterol; 806mg sodium; 78mg calcium; 4mg iron.

DAY 6

Breakfast

3 frozen pancakes, heated and topped with 2 tsp. low-calorie maple syrup
$^1/_2$ medium grapefruit
1 cup nonfat milk

Nutritional Information: 410 calories (9% calories from fat); 3g fat; 15g protein; 63g carbohydrate; 3g dietary fiber; 18mg cholesterol; 842mg sodium.412mg calcium; 1mg iron.

Lunch

Waldorf Salad with Cheese

1 small apple, cored and diced
$^1/_2$ cup celery, chopped
2 cups red cabbage, shredded
2 oz. reduced-fat cheddar cheese, grated
2 tsp. reduced-calorie mayonnaise

In medium bowl, combine apple, celery, cheese and mayonnaise. Top shredded cabbage with salad mixture. Serve with 4 graham crackers ($2^1/_2$-inch squares).

Nutritional Information: 382 calories; 11g fat (23.7% calories from fat); 19g protein; 57g carbohydrate; 9g dietary fiber; 15mg cholesterol; 635mg sodium; 366mg calcium; 3mg iron.

Dinner

Roasted Vegetable Sandwiches

8 slices sourdough bread or 4 pocket pita bread or 4 (2-oz.) rolls
4 oz. low-fat Swiss cheese, sliced

Basil-Yogurt Spread

$^1/_4$ cup plain nonfat yogurt
2 tbsp. reduced-fat mayonnaise
1 tbsp. fresh basil
1 tsp. lemon juice

Whisk together ingredients (can be prepared ahead and refrigerated).

Roasted Vegetables

3 tbsp. balsamic or red wine vinegar
$^1/_4$ cup fresh (or 1 tbsp. dried) basil, chopped
1 red bell pepper, seeded, thinly sliced
1 zucchini, thinly sliced
2 tsp. olive oil
1 yellow summer squash, thinly sliced
1 small red onion, sliced and separated
1 small eggplant, sliced into thin rounds

Preheat oven to 450° F. Blend vinegar, oil and basil. Add vegetables, tossing to coat. Place vegetables in roasting pan and cook, stirring occasionally, until tender and lightly browned, about 30 minutes. Cool vegetables. To assemble sandwiches, spread basil-yogurt mixture on your favorite bread, pita halves or crusty rolls. Top with cheese, fill with veggie mixture and serve. Serves 4.

Nutritional Information: 304 calories (22% calories from fat); 8g fat; 16g protein; 45g carbohydrate; 7g dietary fiber; 13mg cholesterol; 432mg sodium; 377mg calcium; 2mg iron.

DAY 7

Breakfast

3/4 cup raisin-bran cereal
1 cup nonfat milk
1 cup strawberries, sliced
1 slice reduced-calorie wheat bread, toasted and topped with
1 tsp. light margarine

Nutritional Information: 336 calories (12% calories from fat); 5g fat; 16g protein; 64g carbohydrate; 10g dietary fiber; 4mg cholesterol; 591mg sodium; 359mg calcium; 18mg iron.

Lunch

Open-Faced Reuben Sandwich

2 slices reduced-calorie rye bread
1 1/2 oz. lean corned beef, thinly sliced
1/2 oz. reduced-fat Swiss cheese, sliced
black pepper, freshly ground
1/2 tbsp. reduced-fat Thousand Island dressing
1/2 cup sauerkraut, drained

Preheat broiler. Lightly toast bread. To assemble sandwiches, place toast slices onto rack in broiler pan; spread each slice with 1 1/2 tsp. dressing. Top each with 3/4 oz. corned beef, 1/4 cup sauerkraut, another 3/4 oz. corned beef and cheese. Sprinkle evenly with pepper to taste; broil 4 inches from heat for 2 minutes until cheese is melted and lightly browned. Serves 2.

Mustard Yogurt Dip: In small bowl, combine 1/4 cup plain, nonfat yogurt and 2 tbsp. prepared mustard. Serve with 1/2 cup carrot sticks, 1/2 cup cauliflower florets and 1/2 cup sugar-free cherry-flavored gelatin mixed with fruit cocktail per person.

Nutritional Information: 456 calories (23% calories from fat); 12g fat; 24g protein; 67g carbohydrate; 12g dietary fiber; 30mg cholesterol; 1,827mg sodium; 397mg calcium; 6mg iron.

Dinner

Oriental Chicken and Cabbage Salad

1 cup canned, unsalted chicken broth
2 tsp. jalapeno chili, seeded and minced
4 large garlic cloves, minced
4 oz. snow peas, trimmed
1/4 cup fresh cilantro, chopped
3 tbsp. minced fresh (or 1 tsp. ground) ginger
1 1/2 lbs. skinless, boneless chicken breasts, cubed
1/3 cup rice wine vinegar
1 tsp. sesame oil
1 (1-gram) packet sugar substitute
4 1/2 cups red cabbage, sliced

2 cups mushrooms, sliced
2 tbsp. soy sauce, diluted with 2 tbsp. water
$1^1/_2$ cups carrots, grated
1 cup green onions, chopped
$5^1/_2$ cups Napa or green cabbage, sliced

Bring broth to simmer in heavy, large skillet over medium heat. Add chicken and simmer until cooked through, about 7 minutes. Transfer chicken to a bowl to cool. Add snow peas to broth and cook until tender, about 3 minutes. Using slotted spoon, transfer peas to bowl of cold water, then drain and set aside. Boil broth until reduced to $^1/_3$ cup, about 7 minutes. Transfer to bowl; cool. Combine vinegar, chili, cilantro, soy sauce, ginger, garlic, sesame oil and sugar substitute in medium bowl. Add broth and whisk. Place cabbage, mushrooms, carrots and onions in large bowl. Add chicken. Top with dressing and toss to combine. (*Note:* May be made 6 hours ahead. Cover and refrigerate.) For a colorful presentation, serve salad in red cabbage leaves. Serve with $^1/_4$ cup Chinese noodles per person. Serves 6.

Nutritional Information: 402 calories (25% calories from fat); 12g fat; 28g protein; 48g carbohydrate; 6g dietary fiber; 0mg cholesterol; 514mg sodium; 130mg calcium; 4mg iron.

HEALTHY SNACK OPTIONS

30 small pretzel sticks: 90 calories
6 *Lemon-Garlic Pita Chips*: 100 calories (see recipe below)
1 banana-chocolate whip (combine 1 cup fat-free milk, 1 small banana, a squeeze of chocolate syrup and a handful of ice cubes in a blender): 150 calories
3 cups air-popped popcorn sprinkled with 1 tablespoon parmesan cheese: 120 calories
1 *Peanut Butter Biscotti*: 125 calories (see recipe below)
1 mini-bagel with fat-free cream cheese (2 oz.): 145 calories
Snack Plate—25 red grapes, 3 tablespoons feta cheese, 6 crackers: 200 calories
Strawberry Malted Milk Shake: 250 calories (see recipe below)

SNACK RECIPES

Lemon-Garlic Pita Chips

3 (6-inch) pita bread rounds, split in half horizontally
2 teaspoons olive oil
$1^1/_2$ teaspoons lemon pepper
$^1/_4$ teaspoon garlic powder

Preheat oven to 400° F. Cut each pita half into 4 wedges; place on a baking sheet. Drizzle oil evenly over wedges. Combine lemon pepper and garlic powder; sprinkle evenly over wedges. Bake for 5 minutes or until crisp.

Nutritional Information: 146 calories (18% calories from fat); 3g fat; 4g protein; 26g carbohydrate; 1g dietary fiber; 0mg cholesterol; 369mg sodium: 39mg calcium; 1mg iron.

Peanut Butter Biscotti

2 cups all-purpose flour
3/4 cup sugar
3/4 teaspoon baking soda
1/4 teaspoon salt
1/3 cup chunky peanut butter
1 teaspoon vanilla extract
2 large eggs
2 large egg whites
Cooking spray

Preheat oven to 325° F. Lightly spoon flour into dry measuring cups; level with a knife. Combine flour, sugar, baking soda and salt in a large bowl. Combine peanut butter, vanilla, eggs and egg whites in a medium bowl, stirring well with a whisk; add to flour mixture, stirring just until blended. Turn dough out onto a lightly floured surface; shape dough into a 10-inch-long roll. Place roll on a baking sheet coated with cooking spray and flatten to 1-inch thickness. Bake at 325° F for 35 minutes. Remove roll from baking sheet and cool 10 minutes on a wire rack. Reduce oven temperature to 300° F. Cut roll diagonally into 18 (1/2-inch) slices. Place slices, cut sides down, on baking sheet. Bake at 300° F for 20 minutes. Turn cookies over; bake an additional 20 minutes (cookies will be slightly soft in center but will harden as they cool). Remove from baking sheet; cool completely on a wire rack.

Nutritional Information: 125 calories (22% calories from fat); 3g fat; 4g protein; 20g carbohydrate; 1g dietary fiber; 24mg cholesterol; 119mg sodium; 7mg calcium; 1mg iron.

Strawberry Malted Milk Shake

2 cups vanilla low-fat ice cream
1 1/2 cups halved strawberries
1/4 cup skim milk
3 tablespoons malted milk powder
1 tablespoon sugar
Whole strawberries with green caps (optional)

Place first 5 ingredients in a blender, and process until smooth. Garnish with whole strawberries, if desired. Serve immediately.

Nutritional Information: 250 calories (20% calories from fat); 6g fat; 7g protein; 45g carbohydrate; 2g dietary fiber; 16mg cholesterol; 175mg sodium; 213mg calcium: 1mg iron.

Member Survey

Please answer the following questions to help your leader plan your First Place 4 Health meetings so that your needs might be met in this session. Give this form to your leader at the first group meeting.

Name ______________________ Birth date ______________________

Please list those who live in your household.

Name	Relationship	Age

What church do you attend? ______________________

Are you interested in receiving more information about our church?

❒ Yes ❒ No

Occupation ______________________

What talent or area of expertise would you be willing to share with our class?

____

Why did you join First Place 4 Health?

____

With notice, would you be willing to lead a Bible study discussion one week?

❒ Yes ❒ No

Are you comfortable praying out loud? ______________________

If the assistant leader were absent, would you be willing to assist in weighing in members and possibly evaluating the Live It Trackers?

❒ Yes ❒ No

Any other comments:

____

____

____

Personal Weight and Measurement Record

Week	Weight	+ or -	Goal this Session	Pounds to goal
1				
2				
3				
4				
5				
6				
7				
8				
9				
10				
11				
12				

Beginning Measurements

Waist ____________ Hips ____________ Thighs ____________ Chest ____________

Ending Measurements

Waist ____________ Hips ____________ Thighs ____________ Chest ____________

First Place 4 Health
Prayer Partner

4 first place health

BEGIN
WITH CHRIST
Week
2

Seek first his kingdom and his righteousness,
and all these things will be given to you as well.

MATTHEW 6:33

Date: ______________________

Name: ______________________________________

Home Phone: (____)__________________________________

Work Phone: (____)__________________________________

Email: ______________________________________

Personal Prayer Concerns:

____

____

____

____

____

____

____

This form is for prayer requests that are personal to you and your journey in First Place 4 Health. Please complete this form and have it ready to turn in when you at your group meeting.

First Place 4 Health
Prayer Partner

BEGIN WITH CHRIST
Week
3

If you believe, you will receive whatever you ask for in prayer.

MATTHEW 21:22

Date: ______________________

Name: ______________________

Home Phone: (____) ______________________

Work Phone: (____) ______________________

Email: ______________________

Personal Prayer Concerns:

____

____

____

____

____

____

____

This form is for prayer requests that are personal to you and your journey in First Place 4 Health. Please complete this form and have it ready to turn in when you arrive at your group meeting.

First Place 4 Health
Prayer Partner

first place 4 health

BEGIN
WITH CHRIST
Week
4

Whoever has my commands and obeys them, he is the one who loves me.
He who loves me will be loved by my Father,
and I too will love him and show myself to him.

John 14:21

Date: ______________________

Name: ______________________________________

Home Phone: (____) ______________________________

Work Phone: (____) ______________________________

Email: ______________________________________

Personal Prayer Concerns:

____

____

____

____

____

____

____

This form is for prayer requests that are personal to you and your journey in First Place 4 Health. Please complete this form and have it ready to turn in when you arrive at your group meeting.

First Place 4 Health
Prayer Partner

BEGIN
WITH CHRIST
Week
6

No temptation has seized you except what is common to man. And God is faithful, he will not let you be tempted beyond what you can bear. But when you are tempted, he will also provide a way out so that you can stand up under it.

1 Corinthians 10:13

Date: ______________________

Name: ______________________

Home Phone: (____) ______________________

Work Phone: (____) ______________________

Email: ______________________

Personal Prayer Concerns:

____

____

____

____

____

____

____

This form is for prayer requests that are personal to you and your journey in First Place 4 Health. Please complete this form and have it ready to turn in when you arrive at your group meeting.

First Place 4 Health
Prayer Partner

4 first place health

BEGIN
WITH CHRIST
Week
7

Man does not live on bread alone,
but on every word that comes from the mouth of God.

MATTHEW 4:4

Date: ______________________

Name: ______________________

Home Phone: (   ) ______________________

Work Phone: (   ) ______________________

Email: ______________________

Personal Prayer Concerns:

____

____

____

____

____

____

____

This form is for prayer requests that are personal to you and your journey in First Place 4 Health. Please complete this form and have it ready to turn in when you arrive at your group meeting.

First Place 4 Health Prayer Partner

BEGIN
WITH CHRIST
Week
8

Do not conform any longer to the pattern of this world, but be transformed by the renewing of your mind. Then you will be able to test and approve what God's will is—his good, pleasing and perfect will.

Romans 12:2

Date: ______________________

Name: ______________________

Home Phone: (____) ______________________

Work Phone: (____) ______________________

Email: ______________________

Personal Prayer Concerns:

This form is for prayer requests that are personal to you and your journey in First Place 4 Health. Please complete this form and have it ready to turn in when you arrive at your group meeting.

First Place 4 Health
Prayer Partner

first place 4health

BEGIN
WITH CHRIST
Week
9

Do you not know that your body is a temple of the Holy Spirit, who is in you, whom you have received from God? You are not your own; you were bought at a price. Therefore honor God with your body.

1 Corinthians 6:19-20

Date: ______________________

Name: ______________________

Home Phone: (   ) ______________________

Work Phone: (   ) ______________________

Email: ______________________

Personal Prayer Concerns:

____

____

____

____

____

____

____

This form is for prayer requests that are personal to you and your journey in First Place 4 Health. Please complete this form and have it ready to turn in when you arrive at your group meeting.

First Place 4 Health
Prayer Partner

4 first place health

BEGIN
WITH CHRIST
Week
10

Commit to the Lord whatever you do, and your plans will succeed.

Proverbs 16:3

Date: ______________________

Name: ______________________

Home Phone: (____) ______________________

Work Phone: (____) ______________________

Email: ______________________

Personal Prayer Concerns:

____

____

____

____

____

____

____

This form is for prayer requests that are personal to you and your journey in First Place 4 Health. Please complete this form and have it ready to turn in when you arrive at your group meeting.

First Place 4 Health Prayer Partner

first place 4 health

BEGIN WITH CHRIST
Week
11

A new command I give you: Love one another. As I have loved you, so you must love one another. By this all men will know that you are my disciples, if you love one another.

JOHN 13:34-35

Date: ______________________

Name: ______________________________________

Home Phone: (____) ______________________________

Work Phone: (____) ______________________________

Email: ______________________________________

Personal Prayer Concerns:

____

____

____

____

____

____

____

This form is for prayer requests that are personal to you and your journey in First Place 4 Health. Please complete this form and have it ready to turn in when you arrive at your group meeting.

Live It Tracker

Name: ______ My week at a glance: ❑ Great ❑ So-so ❑ Not so great

Date: ______ Week #: ______ Calorie Range: ______ My food goal for next week: ______

Activity Level: None, < 30 min/day, 30-60 min/day, 60+ min/day My activity goal for next week: ______

Scripture Memory Verse: ______

RECOMMENDED DAILY AMOUNT OF FOOD FROM EACH GROUP

Group	Daily Calories							
	1300-1400	1500-1600	1700-1800	1900-2000	2100-2200	2300-2400	2500-2600	2700-2800
Fruits	1.5-2 c.	1.5-2 c.	1.5-2 c.	2-2.5 c.	2- 2.5 c.	2.5- 3.5 c.	3.5- 4.5 c.	3.5- 4.5 c.
Vegetables	1.5-2 c.	2-2.5 c.	2.5-3 c.	2.5-3 c.	3- 3.5 c.	3.5- 4.5 c.	4.5- 5 c.	4.5- 5 c.
Grains	5 oz-eq.	5-6 oz-eq.	6-7 oz-eq.	6-7 oz-eq.	7- 8 oz-eq.	8-9 oz-eq.	9-10 oz-eq.	10-11 oz-eq.
Milk	2- 3 c.	3 c.	3 c.	3 c.	3 c.	3 c.	3 c.	3 c.
Meat & Beans	4 oz-eq.	5 oz-eq.	5- 5.5 oz-eq.	5.5- 6.5 oz-eq.	6.5- 7 oz-eq.	7 -7.5 oz-eq.	7- 7.5 oz-eq.	7.5- 8 oz-eq.
Healthy Oils	4 tsp.	5 tsp.	5 tsp.	6 tsp.	6 tsp.	7 tsp.	8 tsp.	8 tsp.

Day 1

FOOD CHOICES

Breakfast: ______ Lunch: ______

Dinner: ______ Snacks: ______

Group	Fruits	Vegetables	Grains	Milk	Meat & Beans	Healthy Oils
Goal Amount						
Estimate Your Total						
Increase ⇧ or Decrease ⇩?						

PHYSICAL ACTIVITY

Description: ______

Steps/Miles/Minutes: ______

SPIRITUAL ACTIVITY

Description: ______

Day 2

FOOD CHOICES

Breakfast: ______ Lunch: ______

Dinner: ______ Snacks: ______

Group	Fruits	Vegetables	Grains	Milk	Meat & Beans	Healthy Oils
Goal Amount						
Estimate Your Total						
Increase ⇧ or Decrease ⇩?						

PHYSICAL ACTIVITY

Description: ______

Steps/Miles/Minutes: ______

SPIRITUAL ACTIVITY

Description: ______

Day 3

FOOD CHOICES

Breakfast: ______ Lunch: ______

Dinner: ______ Snacks: ______

Group	Fruits	Vegetables	Grains	Milk	Meat & Beans	Healthy Oils
Goal Amount						
Estimate Your Total						
Increase ⇧ or Decrease ⇩?						

PHYSICAL ACTIVITY

Description: ______

Steps/Miles/Minutes: ______

SPIRITUAL ACTIVITY

Description: ______

Day 4

FOOD CHOICES

Breakfast: ______________________ Lunch: ______________________

Dinner: ______________________ Snacks: ______________________

Group	*Fruits*	*Vegetables*	*Grains*	*Milk*	*Meat & Beans*	*Healthy Oils*
Goal Amount						
Estimate Your Total						
Increase ⇧ or Decrease ⇩?						

PHYSICAL ACTIVITY

Description: ______________________

Steps/Miles/Minutes: ______________________

SPIRITUAL ACTIVITY

Description: ______________________

Day 5

FOOD CHOICES

Breakfast: ______________________ Lunch: ______________________

Dinner: ______________________ Snacks: ______________________

Group	*Fruits*	*Vegetables*	*Grains*	*Milk*	*Meat & Beans*	*Healthy Oils*
Goal Amount						
Estimate Your Total						
Increase ⇧ or Decrease ⇩?						

PHYSICAL ACTIVITY

Description: ______________________

Steps/Miles/Minutes: ______________________

SPIRITUAL ACTIVITY

Description: ______________________

Day 6

FOOD CHOICES

Breakfast: ______________________ Lunch: ______________________

Dinner: ______________________ Snacks: ______________________

Group	*Fruits*	*Vegetables*	*Grains*	*Milk*	*Meat & Beans*	*Healthy Oils*
Goal Amount						
Estimate Your Total						
Increase ⇧ or Decrease ⇩?						

PHYSICAL ACTIVITY

Description: ______________________

Steps/Miles/Minutes: ______________________

SPIRITUAL ACTIVITY

Description: ______________________

Day 7

FOOD CHOICES

Breakfast: ______________________ Lunch: ______________________

Dinner: ______________________ Snacks: ______________________

Group	*Fruits*	*Vegetables*	*Grains*	*Milk*	*Meat & Beans*	*Healthy Oils*
Goal Amount						
Estimate Your Total						
Increase ⇧ or Decrease ⇩?						

PHYSICAL ACTIVITY

Description: ______________________

Steps/Miles/Minutes: ______________________

SPIRITUAL ACTIVITY

Description: ______________________

Live It Tracker

Name: ____________ My week at a glance: ❑ Great ❑ So-so ❑ Not so great

Date: ________ Week #: ______ Calorie Range: ________ My food goal for next week: ____________

Activity Level: None, < 30 min/day, 30-60 min/day, 60+ min/day My activity goal for next week: ____________

Scripture Memory Verse: ____________

RECOMMENDED DAILY AMOUNT OF FOOD FROM EACH GROUP

Group	Daily Calories							
	1300-1400	1500-1600	1700-1800	1900-2000	2100-2200	2300-2400	2500-2600	2700-2800
Fruits	1.5-2 c.	1.5-2 c.	1.5-2 c.	2-2.5 c.	2- 2.5 c.	2.5- 3.5 c.	3.5- 4.5 c.	3.5- 4.5 c.
Vegetables	1.5-2 c.	2-2.5 c.	2.5-3 c.	2.5-3 c.	3- 3.5 c.	3.5- 4.5 c.	4.5- 5 c.	4.5- 5 c.
Grains	5 oz-eq.	5-6 oz-eq.	6-7 oz-eq.	6-7 oz-eq.	7- 8 oz-eq.	8-9 oz-eq.	9-10 oz-eq.	10-11 oz-eq.
Milk	2- 3 c.	3 c.	3 c.	3 c.	3 c.	3 c.	3 c.	3 c.
Meat & Beans	4 oz-eq.	5 oz-eq.	5- 5.5 oz-eq.	5.5- 6.5 oz-eq.	6.5- 7 oz-eq.	7 -7.5 oz-eq.	7- 7.5 oz-eq.	7.5- 8 oz-eq.
Healthy Oils	4 tsp.	5 tsp.	5 tsp.	6 tsp.	6 tsp.	7 tsp.	8 tsp.	8 tsp.

Day 1

FOOD CHOICES

Breakfast: ____________ Lunch: ____________

Dinner: ____________ Snacks: ____________

Group	Fruits	Vegetables	Grains	Milk	Meat & Beans	Healthy Oils
Goal Amount						
Estimate Your Total						
Increase ⇧ or Decrease ⇩?						

PHYSICAL ACTIVITY

Description: ____________

Steps/Miles/Minutes: ____________

SPIRITUAL ACTIVITY

Description: ____________

Day 2

FOOD CHOICES

Breakfast: ____________ Lunch: ____________

Dinner: ____________ Snacks: ____________

Group	Fruits	Vegetables	Grains	Milk	Meat & Beans	Healthy Oils
Goal Amount						
Estimate Your Total						
Increase ⇧ or Decrease ⇩?						

PHYSICAL ACTIVITY

Description: ____________

Steps/Miles/Minutes: ____________

SPIRITUAL ACTIVITY

Description: ____________

Day 3

FOOD CHOICES

Breakfast: ____________ Lunch: ____________

Dinner: ____________ Snacks: ____________

Group	Fruits	Vegetables	Grains	Milk	Meat & Beans	Healthy Oils
Goal Amount						
Estimate Your Total						
Increase ⇧ or Decrease ⇩?						

PHYSICAL ACTIVITY

Description: ____________

Steps/Miles/Minutes: ____________

SPIRITUAL ACTIVITY

Description: ____________

Day 4

FOOD CHOICES

Breakfast: ______________________ Lunch: ______________________

Dinner: ______________________ Snacks: ______________________

Group	Fruits	Vegetables	Grains	Milk	Meat & Beans	Healthy Oils
Goal Amount						
Estimate Your Total						
Increase ⇧ or Decrease ⇩?						

PHYSICAL ACTIVITY

Description: ______________________

Steps/Miles/Minutes: ______________________

SPIRITUAL ACTIVITY

Description: ______________________

Day 5

FOOD CHOICES

Breakfast: ______________________ Lunch: ______________________

Dinner: ______________________ Snacks: ______________________

Group	Fruits	Vegetables	Grains	Milk	Meat & Beans	Healthy Oils
Goal Amount						
Estimate Your Total						
Increase ⇧ or Decrease ⇩?						

PHYSICAL ACTIVITY

Description: ______________________

Steps/Miles/Minutes: ______________________

SPIRITUAL ACTIVITY

Description: ______________________

Day 6

FOOD CHOICES

Breakfast: ______________________ Lunch: ______________________

Dinner: ______________________ Snacks: ______________________

Group	Fruits	Vegetables	Grains	Milk	Meat & Beans	Healthy Oils
Goal Amount						
Estimate Your Total						
Increase ⇧ or Decrease ⇩?						

PHYSICAL ACTIVITY

Description: ______________________

Steps/Miles/Minutes: ______________________

SPIRITUAL ACTIVITY

Description: ______________________

Day 7

FOOD CHOICES

Breakfast: ______________________ Lunch: ______________________

Dinner: ______________________ Snacks: ______________________

Group	Fruits	Vegetables	Grains	Milk	Meat & Beans	Healthy Oils
Goal Amount						
Estimate Your Total						
Increase ⇧ or Decrease ⇩?						

PHYSICAL ACTIVITY

Description: ______________________

Steps/Miles/Minutes: ______________________

SPIRITUAL ACTIVITY

Description: ______________________

Live It Tracker

Name: ______________________ My week at a glance: ❑ Great ❑ So-so ❑ Not so great

Date: __________ Week #: ______ Calorie Range: __________ My food goal for next week: ______________

Activity Level: None, < 30 min/day, 30-60 min/day, 60+ min/day My activity goal for next week: ______________

Scripture Memory Verse: ______________________

RECOMMENDED DAILY AMOUNT OF FOOD FROM EACH GROUP

Group	Daily Calories							
	1300-1400	1500-1600	1700-1800	1900-2000	2100-2200	2300-2400	2500-2600	2700-2800
Fruits	1.5-2 c.	1.5-2 c.	1.5-2 c.	2-2.5 c.	2- 2.5 c.	2.5- 3.5 c.	3.5- 4.5 c.	3.5- 4.5 c.
Vegetables	1.5-2 c.	2-2.5 c.	2.5-3 c.	2.5-3 c.	3- 3.5 c.	3.5- 4.5 c.	4.5- 5 c.	4.5- 5 c.
Grains	5 oz-eq.	5-6 oz-eq.	6-7 oz-eq.	6-7 oz-eq.	7- 8 oz-eq.	8-9 oz-eq.	9-10 oz-eq.	10-11 oz-eq.
Milk	2- 3 c.	3 c.	3 c.	3 c.	3 c.	3 c.	3 c.	3 c.
Meat & Beans	4 oz-eq.	5 oz-eq.	5- 5.5 oz-eq.	5.5- 6.5 oz-eq.	6.5- 7 oz-eq.	7 -7.5 oz-eq.	7- 7.5 oz-eq.	7.5- 8 oz-eq.
Healthy Oils	4 tsp.	5 tsp.	5 tsp.	6 tsp.	6 tsp.	7 tsp.	8 tsp.	8 tsp.

Day 1

FOOD CHOICES

Breakfast: ______________ Lunch: ______________

Dinner: ______________ Snacks: ______________

Group	Fruits	Vegetables	Grains	Milk	Meat & Beans	Healthy Oils
Goal Amount						
Estimate Your Total						
Increase ⇧ or Decrease ⇩?						

PHYSICAL ACTIVITY

Description: ______________

Steps/Miles/Minutes: ______________

SPIRITUAL ACTIVITY

Description: ______________

Day 2

FOOD CHOICES

Breakfast: ______________ Lunch: ______________

Dinner: ______________ Snacks: ______________

Group	Fruits	Vegetables	Grains	Milk	Meat & Beans	Healthy Oils
Goal Amount						
Estimate Your Total						
Increase ⇧ or Decrease ⇩?						

PHYSICAL ACTIVITY

Description: ______________

Steps/Miles/Minutes: ______________

SPIRITUAL ACTIVITY

Description: ______________

Day 3

FOOD CHOICES

Breakfast: ______________ Lunch: ______________

Dinner: ______________ Snacks: ______________

Group	Fruits	Vegetables	Grains	Milk	Meat & Beans	Healthy Oils
Goal Amount						
Estimate Your Total						
Increase ⇧ or Decrease ⇩?						

PHYSICAL ACTIVITY

Description: ______________

Steps/Miles/Minutes: ______________

SPIRITUAL ACTIVITY

Description: ______________

Day 4

FOOD CHOICES

Breakfast: ______________________

Lunch: ______________________

Dinner: ______________________

Snacks: ______________________

Group	Fruits	Vegetables	Grains	Milk	Meat & Beans	Healthy Oils
Goal Amount						
Estimate Your Total						
Increase ⇧ or Decrease ⇩?						

PHYSICAL ACTIVITY

Description: ______________________

Steps/Miles/Minutes: ______________________

SPIRITUAL ACTIVITY

Description: ______________________

____

Day 5

FOOD CHOICES

Breakfast: ______________________

Lunch: ______________________

Dinner: ______________________

Snacks: ______________________

Group	Fruits	Vegetables	Grains	Milk	Meat & Beans	Healthy Oils
Goal Amount						
Estimate Your Total						
Increase ⇧ or Decrease ⇩?						

PHYSICAL ACTIVITY

Description: ______________________

Steps/Miles/Minutes: ______________________

SPIRITUAL ACTIVITY

Description: ______________________

____

Day 6

FOOD CHOICES

Breakfast: ______________________

Lunch: ______________________

Dinner: ______________________

Snacks: ______________________

Group	Fruits	Vegetables	Grains	Milk	Meat & Beans	Healthy Oils
Goal Amount						
Estimate Your Total						
Increase ⇧ or Decrease ⇩?						

PHYSICAL ACTIVITY

Description: ______________________

Steps/Miles/Minutes: ______________________

SPIRITUAL ACTIVITY

Description: ______________________

____

Day 7

FOOD CHOICES

Breakfast: ______________________

Lunch: ______________________

Dinner: ______________________

Snacks: ______________________

Group	Fruits	Vegetables	Grains	Milk	Meat & Beans	Healthy Oils
Goal Amount						
Estimate Your Total						
Increase ⇧ or Decrease ⇩?						

PHYSICAL ACTIVITY

Description: ______________________

Steps/Miles/Minutes: ______________________

SPIRITUAL ACTIVITY

Description: ______________________

____

Live It Tracker

Name: ______________________ My week at a glance: ❑ Great ❑ So-so ❑ Not so great

Date: __________ Week #: ______ Calorie Range: __________ My food goal for next week: ______________

Activity Level: None, < 30 min/day, 30-60 min/day, 60+ min/day My activity goal for next week: ______________

Scripture Memory Verse: ____

____

RECOMMENDED DAILY AMOUNT OF FOOD FROM EACH GROUP

Group	*Daily Calories*							
	1300-1400	1500-1600	1700-1800	1900-2000	2100-2200	2300-2400	2500-2600	2700-2800
Fruits	1.5-2 c.	1.5-2 c.	1.5-2 c.	2-2.5 c.	2- 2.5 c.	2.5- 3.5 c.	3.5- 4.5 c.	3.5- 4.5 c.
Vegetables	1.5-2 c.	2-2.5 c.	2.5-3 c.	2.5-3 c.	3- 3.5 c.	3.5- 4.5 c.	4.5- 5 c.	4.5- 5 c.
Grains	5 oz-eq.	5-6 oz-eq.	6-7 oz-eq.	6-7 oz-eq.	7- 8 oz-eq.	8-9 oz-eq.	9-10 oz-eq.	10-11 oz-eq.
Milk	2- 3 c.	3 c.	3 c.	3 c.	3 c.	3 c.	3 c.	3 c.
Meat & Beans	4 oz-eq.	5 oz-eq.	5- 5.5 oz-eq.	5.5- 6.5 oz-eq.	6.5- 7 oz-eq.	7 -7.5 oz-eq.	7- 7.5 oz-eq.	7.5- 8 oz-eq.
Healthy Oils	4 tsp.	5 tsp.	5 tsp.	6 tsp.	6 tsp.	7 tsp.	8 tsp.	8 tsp.

Day 1

FOOD CHOICES

Breakfast: ______________________ Lunch: ______________________

Dinner: ______________________ Snacks: ______________________

Group	*Fruits*	*Vegetables*	*Grains*	*Milk*	*Meat & Beans*	*Healthy Oils*
Goal Amount						
Estimate Your Total						
Increase ⇧ or Decrease ⇩?						

PHYSICAL ACTIVITY

Description: ______________________

Steps/Miles/Minutes: ______________________

SPIRITUAL ACTIVITY

Description: ______________________

____

Day 2

FOOD CHOICES

Breakfast: ______________________ Lunch: ______________________

Dinner: ______________________ Snacks: ______________________

Group	*Fruits*	*Vegetables*	*Grains*	*Milk*	*Meat & Beans*	*Healthy Oils*
Goal Amount						
Estimate Your Total						
Increase ⇧ or Decrease ⇩?						

PHYSICAL ACTIVITY

Description: ______________________

Steps/Miles/Minutes: ______________________

SPIRITUAL ACTIVITY

Description: ______________________

____

Day 3

FOOD CHOICES

Breakfast: ______________________ Lunch: ______________________

Dinner: ______________________ Snacks: ______________________

Group	*Fruits*	*Vegetables*	*Grains*	*Milk*	*Meat & Beans*	*Healthy Oils*
Goal Amount						
Estimate Your Total						
Increase ⇧ or Decrease ⇩?						

PHYSICAL ACTIVITY

Description: ______________________

Steps/Miles/Minutes: ______________________

SPIRITUAL ACTIVITY

Description: ______________________

____

Day 4

FOOD CHOICES

Breakfast: ______________________ Lunch: ______________________

Dinner: ______________________ Snacks: ______________________

Group	Fruits	Vegetables	Grains	Milk	Meat & Beans	Healthy Oils
Goal Amount						
Estimate Your Total						
Increase ⇧ or Decrease ⇩?						

PHYSICAL ACTIVITY

Description: ______________________

Steps/Miles/Minutes: ______________________

SPIRITUAL ACTIVITY

Description: ______________________

____

Day 5

FOOD CHOICES

Breakfast: ______________________ Lunch: ______________________

Dinner: ______________________ Snacks: ______________________

Group	Fruits	Vegetables	Grains	Milk	Meat & Beans	Healthy Oils
Goal Amount						
Estimate Your Total						
Increase ⇧ or Decrease ⇩?						

PHYSICAL ACTIVITY

Description: ______________________

Steps/Miles/Minutes: ______________________

SPIRITUAL ACTIVITY

Description: ______________________

____

Day 6

FOOD CHOICES

Breakfast: ______________________ Lunch: ______________________

Dinner: ______________________ Snacks: ______________________

Group	Fruits	Vegetables	Grains	Milk	Meat & Beans	Healthy Oils
Goal Amount						
Estimate Your Total						
Increase ⇧ or Decrease ⇩?						

PHYSICAL ACTIVITY

Description: ______________________

Steps/Miles/Minutes: ______________________

SPIRITUAL ACTIVITY

Description: ______________________

____

Day 7

FOOD CHOICES

Breakfast: ______________________ Lunch: ______________________

Dinner: ______________________ Snacks: ______________________

Group	Fruits	Vegetables	Grains	Milk	Meat & Beans	Healthy Oils
Goal Amount						
Estimate Your Total						
Increase ⇧ or Decrease ⇩?						

PHYSICAL ACTIVITY

Description: ______________________

Steps/Miles/Minutes: ______________________

SPIRITUAL ACTIVITY

Description: ______________________

____

Live It Tracker

Name: ______________________ My week at a glance: ❑ Great ❑ So-so ❑ Not so great

Date: __________ Week #: ______ Calorie Range: __________ My food goal for next week: ______________

Activity Level: None, < 30 min/day, 30-60 min/day, 60+ min/day My activity goal for next week: ______________

Scripture Memory Verse: ____

____

RECOMMENDED DAILY AMOUNT OF FOOD FROM EACH GROUP

Group	*Daily Calories*							
	1300-1400	1500-1600	1700-1800	1900-2000	2100-2200	2300-2400	2500-2600	2700-2800
Fruits	1.5-2 c.	1.5-2 c.	1.5-2 c.	2-2.5 c.	2- 2.5 c.	2.5- 3.5 c.	3.5- 4.5 c.	3.5- 4.5 c.
Vegetables	1.5-2 c.	2-2.5 c.	2.5-3 c.	2.5-3 c.	3- 3.5 c.	3.5- 4.5 c.	4.5- 5 c.	4.5- 5 c.
Grains	5 oz-eq.	5-6 oz-eq.	6-7 oz-eq.	6-7 oz-eq.	7- 8 oz-eq.	8-9 oz-eq.	9-10 oz-eq.	10-11 oz-eq.
Milk	2- 3 c.	3 c.	3 c.	3 c.	3 c.	3 c.	3 c.	3 c.
Meat & Beans	4 oz-eq.	5 oz-eq.	5- 5.5 oz-eq.	5.5- 6.5 oz-eq.	6.5- 7 oz-eq.	7 -7.5 oz-eq.	7- 7.5 oz-eq.	7.5- 8 oz-eq.
Healthy Oils	4 tsp.	5 tsp.	5 tsp.	6 tsp.	6 tsp.	7 tsp.	8 tsp.	8 tsp.

Day 1

FOOD CHOICES

Breakfast: ______________________ Lunch: ______________________

Dinner: ______________________ Snacks: ______________________

Group	*Fruits*	*Vegetables*	*Grains*	*Milk*	*Meat & Beans*	*Healthy Oils*
Goal Amount						
Estimate Your Total						
Increase ⇧ or Decrease ⇩?						

PHYSICAL ACTIVITY

Description: ______________________

Steps/Miles/Minutes: ______________________

SPIRITUAL ACTIVITY

Description: ______________________

____

Day 2

FOOD CHOICES

Breakfast: ______________________ Lunch: ______________________

Dinner: ______________________ Snacks: ______________________

Group	*Fruits*	*Vegetables*	*Grains*	*Milk*	*Meat & Beans*	*Healthy Oils*
Goal Amount						
Estimate Your Total						
Increase ⇧ or Decrease ⇩?						

PHYSICAL ACTIVITY

Description: ______________________

Steps/Miles/Minutes: ______________________

SPIRITUAL ACTIVITY

Description: ______________________

____

Day 3

FOOD CHOICES

Breakfast: ______________________ Lunch: ______________________

Dinner: ______________________ Snacks: ______________________

Group	*Fruits*	*Vegetables*	*Grains*	*Milk*	*Meat & Beans*	*Healthy Oils*
Goal Amount						
Estimate Your Total						
Increase ⇧ or Decrease ⇩?						

PHYSICAL ACTIVITY

Description: ______________________

Steps/Miles/Minutes: ______________________

SPIRITUAL ACTIVITY

Description: ______________________

____

Day 4

FOOD CHOICES

Breakfast: ____________________ Lunch: ____________________

Dinner: ____________________ Snacks: ____________________

Group	Fruits	Vegetables	Grains	Milk	Meat & Beans	Healthy Oils
Goal Amount						
Estimate Your Total						
Increase ⇧ or Decrease ⇩?						

PHYSICAL ACTIVITY

Description: ____________________

Steps/Miles/Minutes: ____________________

SPIRITUAL ACTIVITY

Description: ____________________

____

Day 5

FOOD CHOICES

Breakfast: ____________________ Lunch: ____________________

Dinner: ____________________ Snacks: ____________________

Group	Fruits	Vegetables	Grains	Milk	Meat & Beans	Healthy Oils
Goal Amount						
Estimate Your Total						
Increase ⇧ or Decrease ⇩?						

PHYSICAL ACTIVITY

Description: ____________________

Steps/Miles/Minutes: ____________________

SPIRITUAL ACTIVITY

Description: ____________________

____

Day 6

FOOD CHOICES

Breakfast: ____________________ Lunch: ____________________

Dinner: ____________________ Snacks: ____________________

Group	Fruits	Vegetables	Grains	Milk	Meat & Beans	Healthy Oils
Goal Amount						
Estimate Your Total						
Increase ⇧ or Decrease ⇩?						

PHYSICAL ACTIVITY

Description: ____________________

Steps/Miles/Minutes: ____________________

SPIRITUAL ACTIVITY

Description: ____________________

____

Day 7

FOOD CHOICES

Breakfast: ____________________ Lunch: ____________________

Dinner: ____________________ Snacks: ____________________

Group	Fruits	Vegetables	Grains	Milk	Meat & Beans	Healthy Oils
Goal Amount						
Estimate Your Total						
Increase ⇧ or Decrease ⇩?						

PHYSICAL ACTIVITY

Description: ____________________

Steps/Miles/Minutes: ____________________

SPIRITUAL ACTIVITY

Description: ____________________

____

Live It Tracker

Name: ______________ My week at a glance: ❑ Great ❑ So-so ❑ Not so great

Date: ______ Week #: ______ Calorie Range: ______ My food goal for next week: ______________

Activity Level: None, < 30 min/day, 30-60 min/day, 60+ min/day My activity goal for next week: ______________

Scripture Memory Verse: ______________

RECOMMENDED DAILY AMOUNT OF FOOD FROM EACH GROUP

Group	*Daily Calories*							
	1300-1400	1500-1600	1700-1800	1900-2000	2100-2200	2300-2400	2500-2600	2700-2800
Fruits	1.5-2 c.	1.5-2 c.	1.5-2 c.	2-2.5 c.	2- 2.5 c.	2.5- 3.5 c.	3.5- 4.5 c.	3.5- 4.5 c.
Vegetables	1.5-2 c.	2-2.5 c.	2.5-3 c.	2.5-3 c.	3- 3.5 c.	3.5- 4.5 c.	4.5- 5 c.	4.5- 5 c.
Grains	5 oz-eq.	5-6 oz-eq.	6-7 oz-eq.	6-7 oz-eq.	7- 8 oz-eq.	8-9 oz-eq.	9-10 oz-eq.	10-11 oz-eq.
Milk	2- 3 c.	3 c.	3 c.	3 c.	3 c.	3 c.	3 c.	3 c.
Meat & Beans	4 oz-eq.	5 oz-eq.	5- 5.5 oz-eq.	5.5- 6.5 oz-eq.	6.5- 7 oz-eq.	7 -7.5 oz-eq.	7- 7.5 oz-eq.	7.5- 8 oz-eq.
Healthy Oils	4 tsp.	5 tsp.	5 tsp.	6 tsp.	6 tsp.	7 tsp.	8 tsp.	8 tsp.

Day 1

FOOD CHOICES

Breakfast: ______________ Lunch: ______________

Dinner: ______________ Snacks: ______________

Group	*Fruits*	*Vegetables*	*Grains*	*Milk*	*Meat & Beans*	*Healthy Oils*
Goal Amount						
Estimate Your Total						
Increase ⇧ or Decrease ⇩?						

PHYSICAL ACTIVITY

Description: ______________

Steps/Miles/Minutes: ______________

SPIRITUAL ACTIVITY

Description: ______________

Day 2

FOOD CHOICES

Breakfast: ______________ Lunch: ______________

Dinner: ______________ Snacks: ______________

Group	*Fruits*	*Vegetables*	*Grains*	*Milk*	*Meat & Beans*	*Healthy Oils*
Goal Amount						
Estimate Your Total						
Increase ⇧ or Decrease ⇩?						

PHYSICAL ACTIVITY

Description: ______________

Steps/Miles/Minutes: ______________

SPIRITUAL ACTIVITY

Description: ______________

Day 3

FOOD CHOICES

Breakfast: ______________ Lunch: ______________

Dinner: ______________ Snacks: ______________

Group	*Fruits*	*Vegetables*	*Grains*	*Milk*	*Meat & Beans*	*Healthy Oils*
Goal Amount						
Estimate Your Total						
Increase ⇧ or Decrease ⇩?						

PHYSICAL ACTIVITY

Description: ______________

Steps/Miles/Minutes: ______________

SPIRITUAL ACTIVITY

Description: ______________

Day 4

FOOD CHOICES

Breakfast: ____________________

Lunch: ____________________

Dinner: ____________________

Snacks: ____________________

Group	*Fruits*	*Vegetables*	*Grains*	*Milk*	*Meat & Beans*	*Healthy Oils*
Goal Amount						
Estimate Your Total						
Increase ⇧ or Decrease ⇩?						

PHYSICAL ACTIVITY

Description: ____________________

Steps/Miles/Minutes: ____________________

SPIRITUAL ACTIVITY

Description: ____________________

____

Day 5

FOOD CHOICES

Breakfast: ____________________

Lunch: ____________________

Dinner: ____________________

Snacks: ____________________

Group	*Fruits*	*Vegetables*	*Grains*	*Milk*	*Meat & Beans*	*Healthy Oils*
Goal Amount						
Estimate Your Total						
Increase ⇧ or Decrease ⇩?						

PHYSICAL ACTIVITY

Description: ____________________

Steps/Miles/Minutes: ____________________

SPIRITUAL ACTIVITY

Description: ____________________

____

Day 6

FOOD CHOICES

Breakfast: ____________________

Lunch: ____________________

Dinner: ____________________

Snacks: ____________________

Group	*Fruits*	*Vegetables*	*Grains*	*Milk*	*Meat & Beans*	*Healthy Oils*
Goal Amount						
Estimate Your Total						
Increase ⇧ or Decrease ⇩?						

PHYSICAL ACTIVITY

Description: ____________________

Steps/Miles/Minutes: ____________________

SPIRITUAL ACTIVITY

Description: ____________________

____

Day 7

FOOD CHOICES

Breakfast: ____________________

Lunch: ____________________

Dinner: ____________________

Snacks: ____________________

Group	*Fruits*	*Vegetables*	*Grains*	*Milk*	*Meat & Beans*	*Healthy Oils*
Goal Amount						
Estimate Your Total						
Increase ⇧ or Decrease ⇩?						

PHYSICAL ACTIVITY

Description: ____________________

Steps/Miles/Minutes: ____________________

SPIRITUAL ACTIVITY

Description: ____________________

____

Live It Tracker

Name: ____________________ My week at a glance: ❑ Great ❑ So-so ❑ Not so great

Date: __________ Week #: ______ Calorie Range: __________ My food goal for next week: __________

Activity Level: None, < 30 min/day, 30-60 min/day, 60+ min/day My activity goal for next week: __________

Scripture Memory Verse: ____________________

RECOMMENDED DAILY AMOUNT OF FOOD FROM EACH GROUP

Group	*Daily Calories*							
	1300-1400	1500-1600	1700-1800	1900-2000	2100-2200	2300-2400	2500-2600	2700-2800
Fruits	1.5-2 c.	1.5-2 c.	1.5-2 c.	2-2.5 c.	2- 2.5 c.	2.5- 3.5 c.	3.5- 4.5 c.	3.5- 4.5 c.
Vegetables	1.5-2 c.	2-2.5 c.	2.5-3 c.	2.5-3 c.	3- 3.5 c.	3.5- 4.5 c.	4.5- 5 c.	4.5- 5 c.
Grains	5 oz-eq.	5-6 oz-eq.	6-7 oz-eq.	6-7 oz-eq.	7- 8 oz-eq.	8-9 oz-eq.	9-10 oz-eq.	10-11 oz-eq.
Milk	2- 3 c.	3 c.	3 c.	3 c.	3 c.	3 c.	3 c.	3 c.
Meat & Beans	4 oz-eq.	5 oz-eq.	5- 5.5 oz-eq.	5.5- 6.5 oz-eq.	6.5- 7 oz-eq.	7 -7.5 oz-eq.	7- 7.5 oz-eq.	7.5- 8 oz-eq.
Healthy Oils	4 tsp.	5 tsp.	5 tsp.	6 tsp.	6 tsp.	7 tsp.	8 tsp.	8 tsp.

Day 1

FOOD CHOICES

Breakfast: __________ Lunch: __________

Dinner: __________ Snacks: __________

Group	*Fruits*	*Vegetables*	*Grains*	*Milk*	*Meat & Beans*	*Healthy Oils*
Goal Amount						
Estimate Your Total						
Increase ⇧ or Decrease ⇩?						

PHYSICAL ACTIVITY

Description: __________

Steps/Miles/Minutes: __________

SPIRITUAL ACTIVITY

Description: __________

Day 2

FOOD CHOICES

Breakfast: __________ Lunch: __________

Dinner: __________ Snacks: __________

Group	*Fruits*	*Vegetables*	*Grains*	*Milk*	*Meat & Beans*	*Healthy Oils*
Goal Amount						
Estimate Your Total						
Increase ⇧ or Decrease ⇩?						

PHYSICAL ACTIVITY

Description: __________

Steps/Miles/Minutes: __________

SPIRITUAL ACTIVITY

Description: __________

Day 3

FOOD CHOICES

Breakfast: __________ Lunch: __________

Dinner: __________ Snacks: __________

Group	*Fruits*	*Vegetables*	*Grains*	*Milk*	*Meat & Beans*	*Healthy Oils*
Goal Amount						
Estimate Your Total						
Increase ⇧ or Decrease ⇩?						

PHYSICAL ACTIVITY

Description: __________

Steps/Miles/Minutes: __________

SPIRITUAL ACTIVITY

Description: __________

FOOD CHOICES

Breakfast: ______________________ Lunch: ______________________

Dinner: ______________________ Snacks: ______________________

Group	Fruits	Vegetables	Grains	Milk	Meat & Beans	Healthy Oils
Goal Amount						
Estimate Your Total						
Increase ⇧ or Decrease ⇩?						

PHYSICAL ACTIVITY

Description: ______________________

Steps/Miles/Minutes: ______________________

SPIRITUAL ACTIVITY

Description: ______________________

____

Day 4

FOOD CHOICES

Breakfast: ______________________ Lunch: ______________________

Dinner: ______________________ Snacks: ______________________

Group	Fruits	Vegetables	Grains	Milk	Meat & Beans	Healthy Oils
Goal Amount						
Estimate Your Total						
Increase ⇧ or Decrease ⇩?						

PHYSICAL ACTIVITY

Description: ______________________

Steps/Miles/Minutes: ______________________

SPIRITUAL ACTIVITY

Description: ______________________

____

Day 5

FOOD CHOICES

Breakfast: ______________________ Lunch: ______________________

Dinner: ______________________ Snacks: ______________________

Group	Fruits	Vegetables	Grains	Milk	Meat & Beans	Healthy Oils
Goal Amount						
Estimate Your Total						
Increase ⇧ or Decrease ⇩?						

PHYSICAL ACTIVITY

Description: ______________________

Steps/Miles/Minutes: ______________________

SPIRITUAL ACTIVITY

Description: ______________________

____

Day 6

FOOD CHOICES

Breakfast: ______________________ Lunch: ______________________

Dinner: ______________________ Snacks: ______________________

Group	Fruits	Vegetables	Grains	Milk	Meat & Beans	Healthy Oils
Goal Amount						
Estimate Your Total						
Increase ⇧ or Decrease ⇩?						

PHYSICAL ACTIVITY

Description: ______________________

Steps/Miles/Minutes: ______________________

SPIRITUAL ACTIVITY

Description: ______________________

____

Day 7

Live It Tracker

Name: ______ My week at a glance: ❑ Great ❑ So-so ❑ Not so great

Date: ______ Week #: ______ Calorie Range: ______ My food goal for next week: ______

Activity Level: None, < 30 min/day, 30-60 min/day, 60+ min/day My activity goal for next week: ______

Scripture Memory Verse: ______

RECOMMENDED DAILY AMOUNT OF FOOD FROM EACH GROUP

Group	*Daily Calories*							
	1300-1400	1500-1600	1700-1800	1900-2000	2100-2200	2300-2400	2500-2600	2700-2800
Fruits	1.5-2 c.	1.5-2 c.	1.5-2 c.	2-2.5 c.	2- 2.5 c.	2.5- 3.5 c.	3.5- 4.5 c.	3.5- 4.5 c.
Vegetables	1.5-2 c.	2-2.5 c.	2.5-3 c.	2.5-3 c.	3- 3.5 c.	3.5- 4.5 c.	4.5- 5 c.	4.5- 5 c.
Grains	5 oz-eq.	5-6 oz-eq.	6-7 oz eq.	6-7 oz-eq.	7- 8 oz-eq.	8-9 oz-eq.	9-10 oz-eq.	10-11 oz-eq.
Milk	2- 3 c.	3 c.	3 c.	3 c.	3 c.	3 c.	3 c.	3 c.
Meat & Beans	4 oz-eq.	5 oz-eq.	5- 5.5 oz-eq.	5.5- 6.5 oz-eq.	6.5- 7 oz-eq.	7 -7.5 oz-eq.	7- 7.5 oz-eq.	7.5- 8 oz-eq.
Healthy Oils	4 tsp.	5 tsp.	5 tsp.	6 tsp.	6 tsp.	7 tsp.	8 tsp.	8 tsp.

Day 1

FOOD CHOICES

Breakfast: ______ Lunch: ______

Dinner: ______ Snacks: ______

Group	*Fruits*	*Vegetables*	*Grains*	*Milk*	*Meat & Beans*	*Healthy Oils*
Goal Amount						
Estimate Your Total						
Increase ⇧ or Decrease ⇩?						

PHYSICAL ACTIVITY

Description: ______

Steps/Miles/Minutes: ______

SPIRITUAL ACTIVITY

Description: ______

Day 2

FOOD CHOICES

Breakfast: ______ Lunch: ______

Dinner: ______ Snacks: ______

Group	*Fruits*	*Vegetables*	*Grains*	*Milk*	*Meat & Beans*	*Healthy Oils*
Goal Amount						
Estimate Your Total						
Increase ⇧ or Decrease ⇩?						

PHYSICAL ACTIVITY

Description: ______

Steps/Miles/Minutes: ______

SPIRITUAL ACTIVITY

Description: ______

Day 3

FOOD CHOICES

Breakfast: ______ Lunch: ______

Dinner: ______ Snacks: ______

Group	*Fruits*	*Vegetables*	*Grains*	*Milk*	*Meat & Beans*	*Healthy Oils*
Goal Amount						
Estimate Your Total						
Increase ⇧ or Decrease ⇩?						

PHYSICAL ACTIVITY

Description: ______

Steps/Miles/Minutes: ______

SPIRITUAL ACTIVITY

Description: ______

Day 4

FOOD CHOICES

Breakfast: ______________________ Lunch: ______________________

Dinner: ______________________ Snacks: ______________________

Group	Fruits	Vegetables	Grains	Milk	Meat & Beans	Healthy Oils
Goal Amount						
Estimate Your Total						
Increase ⇧ or Decrease ⇩?						

PHYSICAL ACTIVITY

Description: ______________________

Steps/Miles/Minutes: ______________________

SPIRITUAL ACTIVITY

Description: ______________________

____

Day 5

FOOD CHOICES

Breakfast: ______________________ Lunch: ______________________

Dinner: ______________________ Snacks: ______________________

Group	Fruits	Vegetables	Grains	Milk	Meat & Beans	Healthy Oils
Goal Amount						
Estimate Your Total						
Increase ⇧ or Decrease ⇩?						

PHYSICAL ACTIVITY

Description: ______________________

Steps/Miles/Minutes: ______________________

SPIRITUAL ACTIVITY

Description: ______________________

____

Day 6

FOOD CHOICES

Breakfast: ______________________ Lunch: ______________________

Dinner: ______________________ Snacks: ______________________

Group	Fruits	Vegetables	Grains	Milk	Meat & Beans	Healthy Oils
Goal Amount						
Estimate Your Total						
Increase ⇧ or Decrease ⇩?						

PHYSICAL ACTIVITY

Description: ______________________

Steps/Miles/Minutes: ______________________

SPIRITUAL ACTIVITY

Description: ______________________

____

Day 7

FOOD CHOICES

Breakfast: ______________________ Lunch: ______________________

Dinner: ______________________ Snacks: ______________________

Group	Fruits	Vegetables	Grains	Milk	Meat & Beans	Healthy Oils
Goal Amount						
Estimate Your Total						
Increase ⇧ or Decrease ⇩?						

PHYSICAL ACTIVITY

Description: ______________________

Steps/Miles/Minutes: ______________________

SPIRITUAL ACTIVITY

Description: ______________________

____

Live It Tracker

Name: ______________________ My week at a glance: ❑ Great ❑ So-so ❑ Not so great

Date: __________ Week #: ______ Calorie Range: __________ My food goal for next week: ______________________

Activity Level: None, < 30 min/day, 30-60 min/day, 60+ min/day My activity goal for next week: ______________________

Scripture Memory Verse: ______________________

RECOMMENDED DAILY AMOUNT OF FOOD FROM EACH GROUP

Group	*Daily Calories*							
	1300-1400	1500-1600	1700-1800	1900-2000	2100-2200	2300-2400	2500-2600	2700-2800
Fruits	1.5-2 c.	1.5-2 c.	1.5-2 c.	2-2.5 c.	2- 2.5 c.	2.5 3.5 c.	3.5- 4.5 c.	3.5- 4.5 c.
Vegetables	1.5-2 c.	2-2.5 c.	2.5-3 c.	2.5-3 c.	3- 3.5 c.	3.5- 4.5 c.	4.5- 5 c.	4.5- 5 c.
Grains	5 oz-eq.	5-6 oz-eq.	6-7 oz-eq.	6-7 oz-eq.	7- 8 oz-eq.	8-9 oz-eq.	9-10 oz-eq.	10-11 oz-eq.
Milk	2- 3 c.	3 c.	3 c.	3 c.	3 c.	3 c.	3 c.	3 c.
Meat & Beans	4 oz-eq.	5 oz-eq.	5- 5.5 oz-eq.	5.5- 6.5 oz-eq.	6.5- 7 oz-eq.	7 -7.5 oz-eq.	7- 7.5 oz-eq.	7.5- 8 oz-eq.
Healthy Oils	4 tsp.	5 tsp.	5 tsp.	6 tsp.	6 tsp.	7 tsp.	8 tsp.	8 tsp.

Day 1

FOOD CHOICES

Breakfast: ______________________ Lunch: ______________________

Dinner: ______________________ Snacks: ______________________

Group	*Fruits*	*Vegetables*	*Grains*	*Milk*	*Meat & Beans*	*Healthy Oils*
Goal Amount						
Estimate Your Total						
Increase ⇧ or Decrease ⇩?						

PHYSICAL ACTIVITY

Description: ______________________

Steps/Miles/Minutes: ______________________

SPIRITUAL ACTIVITY

Description: ______________________

Day 2

FOOD CHOICES

Breakfast: ______________________ Lunch: ______________________

Dinner: ______________________ Snacks: ______________________

Group	*Fruits*	*Vegetables*	*Grains*	*Milk*	*Meat & Beans*	*Healthy Oils*
Goal Amount						
Estimate Your Total						
Increase ⇧ or Decrease ⇩?						

PHYSICAL ACTIVITY

Description: ______________________

Steps/Miles/Minutes: ______________________

SPIRITUAL ACTIVITY

Description: ______________________

Day 3

FOOD CHOICES

Breakfast: ______________________ Lunch: ______________________

Dinner: ______________________ Snacks: ______________________

Group	*Fruits*	*Vegetables*	*Grains*	*Milk*	*Meat & Beans*	*Healthy Oils*
Goal Amount						
Estimate Your Total						
Increase ⇧ or Decrease ⇩?						

PHYSICAL ACTIVITY

Description: ______________________

Steps/Miles/Minutes: ______________________

SPIRITUAL ACTIVITY

Description: ______________________

Day 4

FOOD CHOICES

Breakfast: ______________________

Lunch: ______________________

Dinner: ______________________

Snacks: ______________________

Group	*Fruits*	*Vegetables*	*Grains*	*Milk*	*Meat & Beans*	*Healthy Oils*
Goal Amount						
Estimate Your Total						
Increase ⇧ or Decrease ⇩?						

PHYSICAL ACTIVITY

Description: ______________________

Steps/Miles/Minutes: ______________________

SPIRITUAL ACTIVITY

Description: ______________________

____

Day 5

FOOD CHOICES

Breakfast: ______________________

Lunch: ______________________

Dinner: ______________________

Snacks: ______________________

Group	*Fruits*	*Vegetables*	*Grains*	*Milk*	*Meat & Beans*	*Healthy Oils*
Goal Amount						
Estimate Your Total						
Increase ⇧ or Decrease ⇩?						

PHYSICAL ACTIVITY

Description: ______________________

Steps/Miles/Minutes: ______________________

SPIRITUAL ACTIVITY

Description: ______________________

____

Day 6

FOOD CHOICES

Breakfast: ______________________

Lunch: ______________________

Dinner: ______________________

Snacks: ______________________

Group	*Fruits*	*Vegetables*	*Grains*	*Milk*	*Meat & Beans*	*Healthy Oils*
Goal Amount						
Estimate Your Total						
Increase ⇧ or Decrease ⇩?						

PHYSICAL ACTIVITY

Description: ______________________

Steps/Miles/Minutes: ______________________

SPIRITUAL ACTIVITY

Description: ______________________

____

Day 7

FOOD CHOICES

Breakfast: ______________________

Lunch: ______________________

Dinner: ______________________

Snacks: ______________________

Group	*Fruits*	*Vegetables*	*Grains*	*Milk*	*Meat & Beans*	*Healthy Oils*
Goal Amount						
Estimate Your Total						
Increase ⇧ or Decrease ⇩?						

PHYSICAL ACTIVITY

Description: ______________________

Steps/Miles/Minutes: ______________________

SPIRITUAL ACTIVITY

Description: ______________________

____

Live It Tracker

Name: ______ My week at a glance: ❑ Great ❑ So-so ❑ Not so great

Date: ______ Week #: ______ Calorie Range: ______ My food goal for next week: ______

Activity Level: None, < 30 min/day, 30-60 min/day, 60+ min/day My activity goal for next week: ______

Scripture Memory Verse: ______

RECOMMENDED DAILY AMOUNT OF FOOD FROM EACH GROUP

Group	*Daily Calories*							
	1300-1400	1500-1600	1700-1800	1900-2000	2100-2200	2300-2400	2500-2600	2700-2800
Fruits	1.5-2 c.	1.5-2 c.	1.5-2 c.	2-2.5 c.	2- 2.5 c.	2.5- 3.5 c.	3.5- 4.5 c.	3.5- 4.5 c.
Vegetables	1.5-2 c.	2-2.5 c.	2.5-3 c.	2.5-3 c.	3- 3.5 c.	3.5- 4.5 c.	4.5- 5 c.	4.5- 5 c.
Grains	5 oz-eq.	5-6 oz-eq.	6-7 oz-eq.	6-7 oz-eq.	7- 8 oz-eq.	8-9 oz-eq.	9-10 oz-eq.	10-11 oz-eq.
Milk	2- 3 c.	3 c.	3 c.	3 c.	3 c.	3 c.	3 c.	3 c.
Meat & Beans	4 oz-eq.	5 oz-eq.	5- 5.5 oz-eq.	5.5- 6.5 oz-eq.	6.5- 7 oz-eq.	7 -7.5 oz-eq.	7- 7.5 oz-eq.	7.5- 8 oz-eq.
Healthy Oils	4 tsp.	5 tsp.	5 tsp.	6 tsp.	6 tsp.	7 tsp.	8 tsp.	8 tsp.

Day 1

FOOD CHOICES

Breakfast: ______ Lunch: ______

Dinner: ______ Snacks: ______

Group	*Fruits*	*Vegetables*	*Grains*	*Milk*	*Meat & Beans*	*Healthy Oils*
Goal Amount						
Estimate Your Total						
Increase ⇧ or Decrease ⇩?						

PHYSICAL ACTIVITY

Description: ______

Steps/Miles/Minutes: ______

SPIRITUAL ACTIVITY

Description: ______

Day 2

FOOD CHOICES

Breakfast: ______ Lunch: ______

Dinner: ______ Snacks: ______

Group	*Fruits*	*Vegetables*	*Grains*	*Milk*	*Meat & Beans*	*Healthy Oils*
Goal Amount						
Estimate Your Total						
Increase ⇧ or Decrease ⇩?						

PHYSICAL ACTIVITY

Description: ______

Steps/Miles/Minutes: ______

SPIRITUAL ACTIVITY

Description: ______

Day 3

FOOD CHOICES

Breakfast: ______ Lunch: ______

Dinner: ______ Snacks: ______

Group	*Fruits*	*Vegetables*	*Grains*	*Milk*	*Meat & Beans*	*Healthy Oils*
Goal Amount						
Estimate Your Total						
Increase ⇧ or Decrease ⇩?						

PHYSICAL ACTIVITY

Description: ______

Steps/Miles/Minutes: ______

SPIRITUAL ACTIVITY

Description: ______

Day 4

FOOD CHOICES

Breakfast: ______________________ Lunch: ______________________

Dinner: ______________________ Snacks: ______________________

Group	*Fruits*	*Vegetables*	*Grains*	*Milk*	*Meat & Beans*	*Healthy Oils*
Goal Amount						
Estimate Your Total						
Increase ⇧ or Decrease ⇩?						

PHYSICAL ACTIVITY

Description: ______________________

Steps/Miles/Minutes: ______________________

SPIRITUAL ACTIVITY

Description: ______________________

Day 5

FOOD CHOICES

Breakfast: ______________________ Lunch: ______________________

Dinner: ______________________ Snacks: ______________________

Group	*Fruits*	*Vegetables*	*Grains*	*Milk*	*Meat & Beans*	*Healthy Oils*
Goal Amount						
Estimate Your Total						
Increase ⇧ or Decrease ⇩?						

PHYSICAL ACTIVITY

Description: ______________________

Steps/Miles/Minutes: ______________________

SPIRITUAL ACTIVITY

Description: ______________________

Day 6

FOOD CHOICES

Breakfast: ______________________ Lunch: ______________________

Dinner: ______________________ Snacks: ______________________

Group	*Fruits*	*Vegetables*	*Grains*	*Milk*	*Meat & Beans*	*Healthy Oils*
Goal Amount						
Estimate Your Total						
Increase ⇧ or Decrease ⇩?						

PHYSICAL ACTIVITY

Description: ______________________

Steps/Miles/Minutes: ______________________

SPIRITUAL ACTIVITY

Description: ______________________

Day 7

FOOD CHOICES

Breakfast: ______________________ Lunch: ______________________

Dinner: ______________________ Snacks: ______________________

Group	*Fruits*	*Vegetables*	*Grains*	*Milk*	*Meat & Beans*	*Healthy Oils*
Goal Amount						
Estimate Your Total						
Increase ⇧ or Decrease ⇩?						

PHYSICAL ACTIVITY

Description: ______________________

Steps/Miles/Minutes: ______________________

SPIRITUAL ACTIVITY

Description: ______________________

Live It Tracker

Name: ____________________ My week at a glance: ❑ Great ❑ So-so ❑ Not so great

Date: __________ Week #: ______ Calorie Range: __________ My food goal for next week: ____________________

Activity Level: None, < 30 min/day, 30-60 min/day, 60+ min/day My activity goal for next week: ____________________

Scripture Memory Verse: ____________________

RECOMMENDED DAILY AMOUNT OF FOOD FROM EACH GROUP

Group	*Daily Calories*							
	1300-1400	1500-1600	1700-1800	1900-2000	2100-2200	2300-2400	2500-2600	2700-2800
Fruits	1.5-2 c.	1.5-2 c.	1.5-2 c.	2-2.5 c.	2- 2.5 c.	2.5- 3.5 c.	3.5- 4.5 c.	3.5- 4.5 c.
Vegetables	1.5-2 c.	2-2.5 c.	2.5-3 c.	2.5-3 c.	3- 3.5 c.	3.5- 4.5 c.	4.5- 5 c.	4.5- 5 c.
Grains	5 oz-eq.	5-6 oz-eq.	6-7 oz-eq.	6-7 oz-eq.	7- 8 oz-eq.	8-9 oz-eq.	9-10 oz-eq.	10-11 oz-eq.
Milk	2- 3 c.	3 c.	3 c.	3 c.	3 c.	3 c.	3 c.	3 c.
Meat & Beans	4 oz-eq.	5 oz-eq.	5- 5.5 oz-eq.	5.5- 6.5 oz-eq.	6.5- 7 oz-eq.	7 -7.5 oz-eq.	7- 7.5 oz-eq.	7.5- 8 oz-eq.
Healthy Oils	4 tsp.	5 tsp.	5 tsp.	6 tsp.	6 tsp.	7 tsp.	8 tsp.	8 tsp.

Day 1

FOOD CHOICES

Breakfast: ____________________ Lunch: ____________________

Dinner: ____________________ Snacks: ____________________

Group	*Fruits*	*Vegetables*	*Grains*	*Milk*	*Meat & Beans*	*Healthy Oils*
Goal Amount						
Estimate Your Total						
Increase ⇧ or Decrease ⇩?						

PHYSICAL ACTIVITY

Description: ____________________

Steps/Miles/Minutes: ____________________

SPIRITUAL ACTIVITY

Description: ____________________

Day 2

FOOD CHOICES

Breakfast: ____________________ Lunch: ____________________

Dinner: ____________________ Snacks: ____________________

Group	*Fruits*	*Vegetables*	*Grains*	*Milk*	*Meat & Beans*	*Healthy Oils*
Goal Amount						
Estimate Your Total						
Increase ⇧ or Decrease ⇩?						

PHYSICAL ACTIVITY

Description: ____________________

Steps/Miles/Minutes: ____________________

SPIRITUAL ACTIVITY

Description: ____________________

Day 3

FOOD CHOICES

Breakfast: ____________________ Lunch: ____________________

Dinner: ____________________ Snacks: ____________________

Group	*Fruits*	*Vegetables*	*Grains*	*Milk*	*Meat & Beans*	*Healthy Oils*
Goal Amount						
Estimate Your Total						
Increase ⇧ or Decrease ⇩?						

PHYSICAL ACTIVITY

Description: ____________________

Steps/Miles/Minutes: ____________________

SPIRITUAL ACTIVITY

Description: ____________________

Day 4

FOOD CHOICES

Breakfast: ______________________ Lunch: ______________________

Dinner: ______________________ Snacks: ______________________

Group	Fruits	Vegetables	Grains	Milk	Meat & Beans	Healthy Oils
Goal Amount						
Estimate Your Total						
Increase ⇧ or Decrease ⇩?						

PHYSICAL ACTIVITY

Description: ______________________

Steps/Miles/Minutes: ______________________

SPIRITUAL ACTIVITY

Description: ______________________

Day 5

FOOD CHOICES

Breakfast: ______________________ Lunch: ______________________

Dinner: ______________________ Snacks: ______________________

Group	Fruits	Vegetables	Grains	Milk	Meat & Beans	Healthy Oils
Goal Amount						
Estimate Your Total						
Increase ⇧ or Decrease ⇩?						

PHYSICAL ACTIVITY

Description: ______________________

Steps/Miles/Minutes: ______________________

SPIRITUAL ACTIVITY

Description: ______________________

Day 6

FOOD CHOICES

Breakfast: ______________________ Lunch: ______________________

Dinner: ______________________ Snacks: ______________________

Group	Fruits	Vegetables	Grains	Milk	Meat & Beans	Healthy Oils
Goal Amount						
Estimate Your Total						
Increase ⇧ or Decrease ⇩?						

PHYSICAL ACTIVITY

Description: ______________________

Steps/Miles/Minutes: ______________________

SPIRITUAL ACTIVITY

Description: ______________________

Day 7

FOOD CHOICES

Breakfast: ______________________ Lunch: ______________________

Dinner: ______________________ Snacks: ______________________

Group	Fruits	Vegetables	Grains	Milk	Meat & Beans	Healthy Oils
Goal Amount						
Estimate Your Total						
Increase ⇧ or Decrease ⇩?						

PHYSICAL ACTIVITY

Description: ______________________

Steps/Miles/Minutes: ______________________

SPIRITUAL ACTIVITY

Description: ______________________

Live It Tracker

Name: ______ My week at a glance: ❑ Great ❑ So-so ❑ Not so great

Date: ______ Week #: ______ Calorie Range: ______ My food goal for next week: ______

Activity Level: None, < 30 min/day, 30-60 min/day, 60+ min/day My activity goal for next week: ______

Scripture Memory Verse: ______

RECOMMENDED DAILY AMOUNT OF FOOD FROM EACH GROUP

Group	Daily Calories							
	1300-1400	1500-1600	1700-1800	1900-2000	2100-2200	2300-2400	2500-2600	2700-2800
Fruits	1.5-2 c.	1.5-2 c.	1.5-2 c.	2-2.5 c.	2- 2.5 c.	2.5- 3.5 c.	3.5- 4.5 c.	3.5- 4.5 c.
Vegetables	1.5-2 c.	2-2.5 c.	2.5-3 c.	2.5-3 c.	3- 3.5 c.	3.5- 4.5 c.	4.5- 5 c.	4.5- 5 c.
Grains	5 oz-eq.	5-6 oz-eq.	6-7 oz-eq.	6-7 oz-eq.	7- 8 oz-eq.	8-9 oz-eq.	9-10 oz-eq.	10-11 oz-eq.
Milk	2- 3 c.	3 c.	3 c.	3 c.	3 c.	3 c.	3 c.	3 c.
Meat & Beans	4 oz-eq.	5 oz-eq.	5- 5.5 oz-eq.	5.5- 6.5 oz-eq.	6.5- 7 oz-eq.	7 -7.5 oz-eq.	7- 7.5 oz-eq.	7.5- 8 oz-eq.
Healthy Oils	4 tsp.	5 tsp.	5 tsp.	6 tsp.	6 tsp.	7 tsp.	8 tsp.	8 tsp.

Day 1

FOOD CHOICES

Breakfast: ______ Lunch: ______

Dinner: ______ Snacks: ______

Group	*Fruits*	*Vegetables*	*Grains*	*Milk*	*Meat & Beans*	*Healthy Oils*
Goal Amount						
Estimate Your Total						
Increase ⇧ or Decrease ⇩?						

PHYSICAL ACTIVITY

Description: ______

Steps/Miles/Minutes: ______

SPIRITUAL ACTIVITY

Description: ______

Day 2

FOOD CHOICES

Breakfast: ______ Lunch: ______

Dinner: ______ Snacks: ______

Group	*Fruits*	*Vegetables*	*Grains*	*Milk*	*Meat & Beans*	*Healthy Oils*
Goal Amount						
Estimate Your Total						
Increase ⇧ or Decrease ⇩?						

PHYSICAL ACTIVITY

Description: ______

Steps/Miles/Minutes: ______

SPIRITUAL ACTIVITY

Description: ______

Day 3

FOOD CHOICES

Breakfast: ______ Lunch: ______

Dinner: ______ Snacks: ______

Group	*Fruits*	*Vegetables*	*Grains*	*Milk*	*Meat & Beans*	*Healthy Oils*
Goal Amount						
Estimate Your Total						
Increase ⇧ or Decrease ⇩?						

PHYSICAL ACTIVITY

Description: ______

Steps/Miles/Minutes: ______

SPIRITUAL ACTIVITY

Description: ______

Day 4

FOOD CHOICES

Breakfast: ______________________ Lunch: ______________________

Dinner: ______________________ Snacks: ______________________

Group	*Fruits*	*Vegetables*	*Grains*	*Milk*	*Meat & Beans*	*Healthy Oils*
Goal Amount						
Estimate Your Total						
Increase ⇧ or Decrease ⇩?						

PHYSICAL ACTIVITY

Description: ______________________

Steps/Miles/Minutes: ______________________

SPIRITUAL ACTIVITY

Description: ______________________

Day 5

FOOD CHOICES

Breakfast: ______________________ Lunch: ______________________

Dinner: ______________________ Snacks: ______________________

Group	*Fruits*	*Vegetables*	*Grains*	*Milk*	*Meat & Beans*	*Healthy Oils*
Goal Amount						
Estimate Your Total						
Increase ⇧ or Decrease ⇩?						

PHYSICAL ACTIVITY

Description: ______________________

Steps/Miles/Minutes: ______________________

SPIRITUAL ACTIVITY

Description: ______________________

Day 6

FOOD CHOICES

Breakfast: ______________________ Lunch: ______________________

Dinner: ______________________ Snacks: ______________________

Group	*Fruits*	*Vegetables*	*Grains*	*Milk*	*Meat & Beans*	*Healthy Oils*
Goal Amount						
Estimate Your Total						
Increase ⇧ or Decrease ⇩?						

PHYSICAL ACTIVITY

Description: ______________________

Steps/Miles/Minutes: ______________________

SPIRITUAL ACTIVITY

Description: ______________________

Day 7

FOOD CHOICES

Breakfast: ______________________ Lunch: ______________________

Dinner: ______________________ Snacks: ______________________

Group	*Fruits*	*Vegetables*	*Grains*	*Milk*	*Meat & Beans*	*Healthy Oils*
Goal Amount						
Estimate Your Total						
Increase ⇧ or Decrease ⇩?						

PHYSICAL ACTIVITY

Description: ______________________

Steps/Miles/Minutes: ______________________

SPIRITUAL ACTIVITY

Description: ______________________

let's count our miles!

Join the 100-Mile Club this Session

Can't walk that mile yet? Don't be discouraged! There are exercises you can do to strengthen your body and burn those extra calories. Keep a record on your Live It Tracker of the number of minutes you do these common physical activities, convert those minutes to miles following the chart below, and then mark off each mile you have completed on the chart found on the back of the front cover. Report your miles to your 100-Mile Club representative when you first arrive each week. Remember, you are not competing with anyone else . . . just yourself. Your job is to strive to reach 100 miles before the last meeting in this session. You can do it—just keep on moving!

Walking

slowly, 2 mph	30 min. = 156 cal. = 1 mile
moderately, 3 mph	20 min. = 156 cal. = 1 mile
very briskly, 4 mph	15 min. = 156 cal. = 1 mile
speed walking	10 min. = 156 cal. = 1 mile
up stairs	13 min. = 159 cal. = 1 mile

Running/Jogging

10 min. = 156 cal. = 1 mile

Cycling Outdoors

slowly, <10 mph	20 min. = 156 cal. = 1 mile
light effort, 10-12 mph	12 min. = 156 cal. = 1 mile
moderate effort, 12-14 mph.	10 min. = 156 cal. = 1 mile
vigorous effort, 14-16 mph	7.5 min. = 156 cal. = 1 mile
very fast, 16-19 mph	6.5 min. = 152 cal. = 1 mile

Sports Activities

Playing tennis (singles)	10 min. = 156 cal. = 1 mile
Swimming	
light to moderate effort	11 min. = 152 cal. = 1 mile
fast, vigorous effort	7.5 min. = 156 cal. = 1 mile
Softball	15 min. = 156 cal. = 1 mile
Golf	20 min. = 156 cal = 1 mile
Rollerblading	6.5 min. = 152 cal. = 1 mile
Ice skating	11 min. = 152 cal. = 1 mile

Jumping rope	7.5 min. = 156 cal. = 1 mile
Basketball	12 min. = 156 cal. = 1 mile
Soccer (casual)	15 min. = 159 cal. = 1 mile

Around the House

Mowing grass	22 min. = 156 cal. = 1 mile
Mopping, sweeping, vacuuming	19.5 min. = 155 cal. = 1 mile
Cooking	40 min. =160 cal. = 1 mile
Gardening	19 min. = 156 cal. = 1 mile
Housework (general)	35 min. = 156 cal. = 1 mile
Ironing	45 min. = 153 cal. = 1 mile
Raking leaves	25 min. = 150 cal. = 1 mile
Washing car	23 min. = 156 cal. = 1 mile
Washing dishes	45 min. = 153 cal. = 1 mile

At the Gym

Stair machine	8.5 min. = 155 cal. = 1 mile
Stationary bike	
slowly, 10 mph	30 min. = 156 cal. = 1 mile
moderately, 10-13 mph	15 min. = 156 cal. = 1 mile
vigorously, 13-16 mph	7.5 min. = 156 cal. = 1 mile
briskly, 16-19 mph	6.5 min. = 156 cal. = 1 mile
Elliptical trainer	12 min. = 156 cal. = 1 mile
Weight machines (used vigorously)	13 min. = 152 cal.=1 mile
Aerobics	
low impact	15 min. = 156 cal. = 1 mile
high impact	12 min. = 156 cal. = 1 mile
water	20 min. = 156 cal. = 1 mile
Pilates	15 min. = 156 cal. = 1 mile
Raquetball (casual)	15 min. = 159 cal. = 1 mile
Stretching exercises	25 min. = 150 cal. = 1 mile
Weight lifting (also works for weight machines used moderately or gently)	30 min. = 156 cal. = 1 mile

Family Leisure

Playing piano	37 min. = 155 cal. = 1 mile
Jumping rope	10 min. = 152 cal. = 1 mile
Skating (moderate)	20 min. = 152 cal. = 1 mile
Swimming	
moderate	17 min. = 156 cal. = 1 mile
vigorous	10 min. = 148 cal. = 1 mile
Table tennis	25 min. = 150 cal. = 1 mile
Walk/run/play with kids	25 min. = 150 cal. = 1 mile